A-Z Midwifery

T0195341

For Elsevier
Senior Content Strategist: Alison Taylor
Content Development Specialists: Veronika Watkins and Katie Golsby
Project Manager: Julie Taylor
Designer: Paula Catalano

A-Z Midwifery

Diane M. Fraser, BEd MPhil PhD MTD RM RGN
Formerly Professor of Midwifery and Head of Academic Division of Midwifery, Faculty of Medicine and Health Sciences, University of Nottingham, Queen's Medical Centre, Nottingham, UK

Margaret A. Cooper, BA RGN RM MTD
Formerly Pre-registration Midwifery Programme Director, Academic Division of Midwifery, Faculty of Medicine and Health Sciences, University of Nottingham, Queen's Medical Centre, Nottingham, UK

Text selection and additional material
Mandy Galloway, for
The Practising Midwife

ELSEVIER

Edinburgh   London   New York   Oxford   Philadelphia
St Louis   Sydney   Toronto   2018

ELSEVIER

ISBN 978-0-7020-7587-2

ELSEVIER your source for books, journals and multimedia in the health sciences

www.elsevierhealth.com

  Working together to grow libraries in developing countries

The publisher's policy is to use **paper manufactured from sustainable forests**

www.elsevier.com • www.bookaid.org

Printed in China

Acknowledgements

Elsevier material been extracted or adapted from *Mayes Midwifery*, 14th Edition (ISBN-13: 9780702052330), *Myles Textbook for Midwives* 15th Edition (ISBN-13: 978-0443069390), *Survival Guide to Midwifery*, 2nd Edition (ISBN-13: 9780702045868), and *The British Liver Trust*.

Figure credits:

Figures 1–6, 8–12, 14–19, 21–29 and 31–39 are extracted from *Myles Textbook for Midwives*, 15th Edition.

Figures 7, 20 and 30 are extracted from *Myles Textbook for Midwives*, 16th Edition.

Figure 13 is reproduced with permission from Gwen Shockey/Science Photo Library.

The following entries have been prepared by *The Practising Midwife*:

ABO incompatibility; AIDS; Alcohol consumption; Anaphylaxis; Anticoagulation Therapy; Anxiety; Arrhythmias, cardiac; Bandl's Ring; Body Mass Index (BMI); Bradycardia; Breastfeeding; Breech Presentation; Burns Marshall Method; Chorioamnionitis; Coombs' Test; Conjoined twins; Constipation; Depression; Disseminated Intravascular Coagulation (DIC); Dystocia; Entonox; Female Genital Mutilation; Ferguson Reflex; Fetal Alcohol Syndrome (FAS); Fontanelles; German Measles; Gestational Diabetes; Healthcare associated infections; Haemorrhagic disease of the newborn; Hepatitis; Herpes; HIV; Infertility; Influenza/Influenza vaccination; Instrumental Delivery; Forceps; Ventouse method; Intrauterine Death; Jaundice; Karyotyping; Kernicterus (bilirubin toxicity); Ketoacidosis; Ketonuria; Kidney disease; Kleihauer Test; Klinefelter syndrome; Laboratory results; McRoberts manoeuvre; Needlestick/Sharps Injury; Neonatal intensive care unit (NICU); Neonatal specialist care; Neural tube defects; Nosocomial infections; Obesity; Pain; Prematurity/Preterm birth; Prostaglandins; Pyrexia; Quadruplets; Quickening; Rubella; Sepsis; Smoking in pregnancy; Stillbirth; Symphysiotomy; Tachycardia; TENS; Vaginal birth after caesarean (VBAC); Vaginal seeding; Wharton's jelly; Zika virus.

Introduction

Modern midwifery education is both exciting and challenging, and finding reliable, quality assured, current information can be tough for many students. To help with this ongoing need, Elsevier and *The Practising Midwife* have teamed together to present you with this brand-new resource which is designed to provide a complete package of 'quick reference', up-to-date information, arranged in an easy-to-use A–Z format.

Taking easily assimilated extracts of content originally prepared by Diane Fraser and Margaret Cooper, leading figures in UK Midwifery Education and Practice, the editorial team at *The Practising Midwife* identified and supplied additional entries to provide an extensive collection of topics covering all the basic midwifery terms, ranging from anatomy and physiology to current policy and practice. Updated artwork – with many illustrations taken from *Myles Textbook for Midwives* – helps complete the picture.

We hope that you enjoy using the *A–Z Midwifery* and invite readers to make suggestions for additions and improvements for future editions.

Good luck with your studies and enjoy your professional life – it is a great privilege to be part of such a wonderful profession!

Elsevier and *The Practising Midwife*
2017

ABO incompatibility

ABO incompatibility (isoimmunization) usually occurs when the mother is blood group O and the baby is group A or, less often, group B. Individuals with type O blood develop antibodies throughout life from exposure to antigens in food, gram-negative bacteria or blood transfusion. By the time of the first pregnancy, they may already have high levels of serum anti-A and anti-B antibodies, which can attack the red blood cells in the fetus resulting in haemolysis (haemolytic disease of the newborn). Severe haemolysis is less common with ABO incompatibility than with rhesus D incompatibility, but the midwife should be alert to the possibility in women with group O blood.

ABO incompatibility usually manifests at less than 36 hours of age, although it may not become obvious until after 48 hours. Diagnostic findings include jaundice, pallor and enlarged liver and spleen (hepatosplenomegaly).

Babies diagnosed and treated for ABO incompatibility need to be closely observed for signs of late anaemia which may occur due to ongoing haemolysis by antibodies that may persist in the baby's circulation for several weeks. Symptoms include lethargy, pallor and poor feeding history. Folate and iron may be prescribed to encourage red blood cell production, but it is not unusual for a baby to develop a severe anaemia requiring transfusion. It can be helpful for the midwife to provide continuity of care up to 28 days.

Further reading

Canadian Paediatric Society, 2007, reaffirmed 2016. Guidelines for detection, management and prevention of hyperbilirubinemia in term and late preterm newborn infants. http://www.cps.ca/documents/position/hyperbilirubinemia-newborn.

Gandhi, A., 2016. Haemolytic disease of the fetus and newborn. (Professional reference.) https://patient.info/doctor/haemolytic-disease-of-the-fetus-and-newborn.

National Institute for Health and Care Excellence, 2010, updated May 2016. Jaundice in newborn babies under 28 days. Clinical guideline 98. https://www.nice.org.uk/guidance/cg98.

AIDS See HIV, Sexually transmitted infections.

Alcohol consumption

Drinking in pregnancy can lead to long-term harm to the unborn baby, and the more alcohol is consumed, the greater the risk. New guidelines on drinking were proposed by the UK Government and published in January 2016. They state that if pregnant or planning a pregnancy, the safest approach is not to drink alcohol at all, to keep risks to the baby to a minimum.

In the UK many women either do not drink alcohol (19%) or stop drinking during pregnancy (40%). The risk of harm to the baby is likely to be low if the woman has drunk only small amounts of alcohol before she knew she was pregnant or during pregnancy.

Women who find out they are pregnant after already having drunk during pregnancy should avoid further drinking, but in most cases it is unlikely that their baby has been affected.

Alcohol can have a wide range of impacts on the unborn baby, known under the umbrella term of fetal alcohol spectrum disorders. Drinking heavily during pregnancy can cause the baby to develop fetal alcohol syndrome, a serious condition causing:

+ restricted growth
+ facial abnormalities
+ learning and behavioural disorders, which may be lifelong

The risks of low birth weight, preterm birth and being small for gestational age may increase in mothers drinking more than 1–2 units/day in pregnancy. It is important that women do not underestimate their actual consumption (see What is a unit?)following.

What is a unit?

+ 10 mL or 8 g of pure alcohol (ethanol)
+ One 25-mL single measure of whisky (alcohol by volume [ABV] 40%)
+ One-third of a pint of beer (ABV 5%–6%)
+ Half of a standard (175 mL) glass of wine (ABV 12%)

More examples

+ Beer, cider, lager (5%) bottle, 330 mL = 1.7 units
+ Beer, cider, lager (5%) pint, 568 mL = 2.8 units
+ Spirits (38%–40%) small measure, 25 mL = 1 unit
+ Sherry, port (17.5%–20%) standard measure, 50 mL = 0.9–1 unit
+ Red/white/rose wine (11%–14%) small glass, 125 mL = 1.4–1.75 units
+ Red/white/rose wine (11%–14%) standard glass, 175 mL = 1.9–2.5 units

+ Red/white/rose wine (11%–14%) large glass, 250 mL = 2.8–3.5 units

Calculation

No. of units = strength (ABV%) × volume (mL) ÷ 1000, e.g., a pint of Stella Artois = (5.2 × 568 ÷ 1000) = 2.95 units

In more general terms, the guidelines propose that for both men and women:

+ It is safest not to regularly drink more than 14 units per week.
+ If drinking this amount, it should be spread over 3 days or more. One or two heavy drinking sessions increases the risks of death from long-term illnesses, accidents and injuries.
+ The risk of developing a range of illnesses, e.g., cancers of the mouth, throat and breast, heart disease, liver disease and epilepsy, increases with any amount drunk on a regular basis.
+ A good way to cut down the amount of alcohol consumed is to have several drink-free days each week.

Some people, such as young adults, older people, those with low body weight, those with other health problems and those taking medicines or other drugs, are more likely to be affected more by alcohol and should be more careful of their level of drinking on one occasion (commonly known as binge drinking).

Further reading

Drinkaware. https://www.drinkaware.co.uk/.

Health and Social Care Information Centre, 2015. Statistics on alcohol, England. http://content.digital.nhs.uk/catalogue/PUB17712/alc-eng-2015-rep.pdf.

UK Chief Medical Officers' Alcohol Guidelines Review. Summary of the proposed new guidelines. https://www.gov.uk/government/uploads/system/uploads/attachment_data/file/489795/summary.pdf.

Anaemia

Anaemia is a deficiency in the quality or quantity of red blood cells, resulting in the reduced oxygen-carrying capacity of the blood. In the UK, the National Institute for Health and Clinical Excellence (NICE) recommends that routine iron supplementation in pregnancy is *not* necessary but that it is warranted when haemoglobin levels are lower than 11 g/dL at first contact or 10.5 g/dL at 28 weeks.

The World Health Organization (WHO) has warned of the risks of anaemia to pregnant women, and estimates that 42% of pregnant women worldwide are anaemic. At least half of this burden is assumed to be due to iron deficiency with the rest due to conditions such as folate, vitamin B12 or vitamin A deficiency, chronic inflammation, parasitic infections and inherited disorders. The highest rates of anaemia occur in Africa and the Indian subcontinent.

Types of anaemia

- Iron deficiency anaemia
- Folic acid deficiency anaemia
- Haemoglobinopathies, including sickle cell and thalassaemia
- Anaemia as a result of blood loss or secondary to infection
- Aplastic anaemia (rare in pregnancy)

Effects on pregnancy and childbirth

- Undermines the woman's general health
- Lowers resistance to infection
- Exacerbates minor disorders of pregnancy, e.g., digestive problems
- In severe cases, may cause intrauterine hypoxia
- Increases severity of antepartum and postpartum haemorrhage
- Increases risk of
  - thromboembolic disorders
  - postnatal depression
  - maternal mortality

Signs and symptoms

- Pallor of mucous membranes
- Tiredness, dizziness, fainting
- Dyspnoea on exertion
- Palpitation
- Oedema
- Digestive upsets, loss of appetite

Iron deficiency anaemia

Investigations include haemoglobin level, mean corpuscular volume, packed cell volume, total iron binding capacity and serum ferritin.

Management

Where iron deficiency anaemia has been confirmed, oral iron 120–140 mg daily may be given as

- ferrous sulphate 200 mg twice daily
- ferrous gluconate 600 mg twice daily

In severe anaemia, iron by intramuscular injection may be required.

Folic acid deficiency anaemia

Folic acid is necessary for the formation of nuclei in all body cells. In pregnancy, when cells proliferate, deficiency may occur unless intake is increased.

Management

All pregnant women and those intending to become pregnant are recommended to take 0.4–4 mg folic acid daily until term.

Further reading

Centers for Disease Control and Prevention, 2015. Folic acid— recommendations. http://www.cdc.gov/ncbddd/folicacid/ recommendations.html.

Knott, L., 2013. Folate deficiency. (Professional reference.) http:// patient.info/doctor/folate-deficiency.

NICE, 2008, updated November 2014. Maternal and child nutrition. Public health guideline PH11. https://www.nice.org.uk/guidance/ ph11.

WHO, 2016. WHO recommendations on antenatal care for a positive pregnancy experience. http://www.who.int/nutrition/ publications/guidelines/antenatalcare-pregnancy-positive-experience/en/.

Anaphylactic syndrome of pregnancy

This rare but potentially catastrophic condition occurs when amniotic fluid enters the maternal pulmonary circulation via the uterine sinuses of the placental site. The presence of amniotic fluid triggers an anaphylactoid response. Although also known as amniotic fluid embolism, the term embolus is a misnomer.

The body responds in two phases:

- The initial phase is one of pulmonary vasospasm causing hypoxia.
- The second phase sees the development of left ventricular failure with haemorrhage, coagulation disorder and further uncontrollable haemorrhage.

Amniotic fluid embolism can occur at any time but the most common is during labour and its immediate aftermath. It should be suspected in cases of sudden collapse or incontrollable bleeding. Maternal and fetal/ neonatal mortality and morbidity are high. However, with immediate resuscitation in a well-equipped hospital, it is no longer the universally fatal condition of the past.

Management is with resuscitation (ABC—airway, breathing, circulation), immediate management of coagulopathy, aggressive treatment of uterine atony with oxytocics, ergometrine and prostaglandins, and adjunctive techniques, e.g., packing, tamponade or Rusch balloons. If bleeding cannot be controlled, emergency hysterectomy is indicated and may be life-saving.

Further reading

Anaphylaxis Campaign Helpline. Tel.: +44-(0)1252-542029 http://www.anaphylaxis.org.uk.

Payne, J., 2015. Amniotic fluid embolism. (Professional reference.) http://patient.info/doctor/amniotic-fluid-embolism.

UK Resuscitation Council. http://www.resus.org.uk.

Anaphylaxis

A severe systemic allergic reaction involving both circulatory and respiratory changes, often accompanied by skin changes. It can be fatal if not diagnosed, addressed and treated quickly and correctly. The Resuscitation Council defines anaphylaxis by the following **ABCDE** criteria:

*   life-threatening **a**irway and/or **b**reathing and/or **c**irculation problems
*   skin and/or mucosal changes (flushing, urticaria, angioedema) in up to 80% of cases
*   sudden onset and rapid progression of symptoms
*   diagnosis is further supported if the patient has been **e**xposed to a known allergen

Treatment

Early intramuscular (IM) injection with adrenaline is the treatment of choice. Give adrenaline IM at the midpoint of the anterolateral thigh (through light clothing if necessary). Repeat after 5 mins if condition has not improved or is getting worse. *Always follow the latest guidance.* The adrenaline dosage for anaphylaxis is:

*   adult or child >12 years: 0.5 mL of 1:1000 solution (500 µg)
*   child 6–12 years: 0.3 mL of 1:1000 solution (300 µg)
*   child under 6 years: 0.15 mL of 1:1000 solution (150 µg)

Individuals at risk of anaphylaxis need to carry adrenaline at all times and need to be instructed in advance when and how to inject it. The latest guidance is that:

+ Two injection devices should be carried at all times to treat symptoms until medical assistance is available; if, after the first injection, the individual does not start to feel better, the second injection should be given 5 to 15 minutes after the first.
+ An ambulance should be called after every administration, even if symptoms improve.
+ The individual should lie down with legs raised (unless they have breathing difficulties, when they should sit up) and, if possible, should not be left alone.

Auto-injection devices should be prescribed by brand name as instructions for use vary between devices, and it is essential that the individual has the type of injector that they have been instructed how to use.

The Anaphylaxis Campaign website has guidance for health professionals on how to use these devices.

Further reading/resources

Anaphylaxis Campaign. http://www.anaphylaxis.org.uk/living-with-anaphylaxis/strategies-for-living-with-allergy/care-and-medication/.
Resuscitation Council. https://www.resus.org.uk/anaphylaxis/emergency-treatment-of-anaphylactic-reactions/.

Antenatal care

Antenatal care is the routine care that all healthy women can expect to receive during their pregnancy.

The aim is to monitor the progress of pregnancy in order to support maternal health and normal fetal development. The midwife critically evaluates the physical, psychological and sociological effects of pregnancy on the woman and her family by:

+ Developing a partnership with the woman
+ Providing a holistic approach to the woman's care that meets her individual needs
+ Promoting awareness of public health issues for the woman and her family
+ Exchanging information with the woman and her family and enabling them to make informed choices about pregnancy and birth
+ Being an advocate for the woman and her family during pregnancy, supporting her right to choose care that is appropriate for her own needs and those of her family

- Recognizing the complications of pregnancy and appropriately referring the woman within the multidisciplinary team
- Assisting the woman and her family in their preparations to meet the demands of birth, and making a birth plan
- Assisting the woman in making an informed choice about methods of infant feeding and giving appropriate and sensitive advice to support her decision
- Offering education for parenthood within a planned programme or on an individual basis
- Working in partnership with other pertinent organizations

The National Institute for Health and Care Excellence (NICE) (2008) recommends pregnant women should be offered information based on current available evidence , together with support, to enable them to make informed decisions about their care, including where they will be seen and who will undertake their care.

Ongoing antenatal care (Fig. 1)

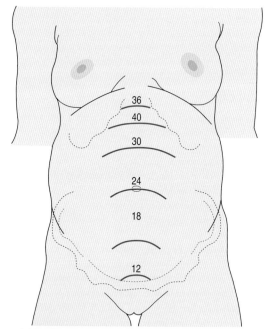

Fig. 1 Fundal heights at various weeks of pregnancy.

16 weeks

- Review, discuss and document results of screening tests undertaken at initial assessment
- Investigate a haemoglobin level below 11 g/dL and consider iron supplementation (see Anaemia)
- Measure blood pressure
- Urinalysis for proteinuria
- Information exchange and review of care plan

18–20 weeks

- Ultrasound scan to detect fetal anomalies

25 weeks

- Measure fundal height
- Measure blood pressure
- Urinalysis for proteinuria
- Information exchange and review of care plan

28 weeks

- Offer repeat screening for anaemia and atypical red-cell alloantibodies
- Investigate a haemoglobin level below 10.5 g/dL and consider iron supplementation (see Anaemia)
- Offer anti-D to rhesus-negative women
- Measure fundal height
- Measure blood pressure
- Urinalysis for proteinuria
- Information exchange and review of care plan

31 weeks (nulliparous women)

- Measure fundal height
- Measure blood pressure
- Urinalysis for proteinuria
- Review, discuss and document results of screening tests undertaken at 28-week assessment
- Information exchange and review of care plan

34 weeks

- Offer a second dose of anti-D to rhesus-negative women (some Trusts only offer one dose of anti-D at 28–30 weeks)
- Measure fundal height
- Measure blood pressure
- Urinalysis for proteinuria

- Multiparous women: review, discuss and document results of screening tests undertaken at 28-week assessment
- Information exchange and review of care plan

36 weeks

- Measure blood pressure
- Urinalysis for proteinuria
- Measure fundal height
- Check presentation of fetus: refer to obstetrician if breech
- Information exchange and review of care plan

38 weeks

- Measure blood pressure
- Urinalysis for proteinuria
- Measure fundal height
- Information exchange and review of care plan

40 weeks (nulliparous women)

- Measure blood pressure
- Urinalysis for proteinuria
- Measure fundal height
- Information exchange and review of care plan

41 weeks

- Measure blood pressure
- Urinalysis for proteinuria
- Measure fundal height
- Information exchange and review of care plan
- Offer a membrane sweep
- Offer induction of labour

Further reading

NICE, 2008, updated March 2016. Antenatal care for uncomplicated pregnancies. Clinical guideline 62. https://www.nice.org.uk/guidance/cg62.

Antenatal examination

An integral part of antenatal care is the physical examination of the pregnant woman. Prior to examination, her consent and comfort are primary considerations.

The examination should include the following components.

Weight

+ All women should be weighed at booking, or asked their pre-pregnant weight.
+ If it is within the normal body mass index (BMI) range, repeated weighing is not recommended.
+ Women with a BMI of >30 kg/m^2 or <18 kg/m^2 should be carefully monitored and offered nutritional counselling.

Blood pressure

Blood pressure (BP) is taken to ascertain normality and provide a baseline reading for comparison throughout pregnancy.

+ Systolic BP may be falsely elevated if the woman is nervous or anxious; a full bladder can cause an increase in BP.
+ The woman should be seated or resting in a lateral position on the couch when BP is taken.
+ A systolic BP of 140 mmHg or diastolic pressure of 90 mmHg at booking is indicative of hypertension and will need careful monitoring throughout pregnancy.

Urinalysis

+ At the first visit a midstream urine (MSU) specimen should be sent to the laboratory for culture to exclude asymptomatic bacteriuria.
+ Urinalysis for proteinuria is performed at every visit.

Blood tests

The following blood tests are performed at the initial assessment:

+ ABO blood group and rhesus (Rh) factor
+ full blood count
+ Venereal Disease Research Laboratory (VDRL) test
+ Human immunodeficiency virus (HIV) antibodies
+ rubella immune status (not at all Trusts)
+ hepatitis B screening
+ investigations for other blood disorders, e.g., sickle cell disease and/or thalassaemia in women and their partners of some ethnic groups

Abdominal examination

Abdominal examination is carried out to establish and affirm that fetal growth is consistent with gestational age during the progression of pregnancy.

Auscultation

Routine auscultation of the fetal heart is not recommended unless requested by the mother. Using a Pinard stethoscope, the midwife should count beats per minute, which should be in the range of 110–160 beats/min. The midwife should take the woman's pulse at the same time to be able to distinguish between the two.

Using ultrasound equipment, e.g., Sonicaid or Doppler enables the woman to hear the fetal heartbeat.

Antenatal screening

Tests for fetal abnormality

There are two types of test for fetal anomaly.

- Screening tests
- Diagnostic tests

Screening for fetal abnormality

Screening tests aim to identify a proportion of individuals who have the highest chance of a named disorder. This makes it possible to target further investigations towards those with the best indication. Women who undergo screening tests will be classified as above or below an action limit, whereby they are recalled and offered follow-up procedures.

Diagnosis for fetal abnormality

Diagnostic tests are performed to confirm or rule out the presence of a particular abnormality.

Before offering screening/diagnostic tests it is essential to obtain informed consent. The following should be discussed:

- the purpose of the procedure
- all risks and benefits that may reasonably be expected
- details of future treatments that could arise as a consequence of testing
- disclosure of all appropriate techniques that may be advantageous
- the option of refusing any tests
- the offer to answer any queries

Ultrasound screening for fetal anomalies

Ultrasound screening for fetal anomalies should be routinely offered, normally between 18 weeks and 20 weeks 6 days. Guidance from the UK's National Institute for Health and Care Excellence (NICE) (2008) states: 'At first contact with a healthcare professional, women should be given information about the purpose and implications of the anomaly scan to enable them to make an informed choice as to whether or not to have the scan: the purpose is to identify fetal anomalies and allow:

+ reproductive choice (termination of pregnancy)
+ parents to prepare (for any treatment/disability/palliative care/termination of pregnancy)
+ managed birth in a specialist centre
+ intrauterine therapy.'

If an anomaly is detected, the woman should be informed of the findings to enable them to make an informed choice about whether or not they wish to continue with the pregnancy or have a termination of pregnancy.

The routine anomaly scan should include:

+ Fetal echocardiography (routine nuchal translucency screening for cardiac anomalies is not recommended)
+ Neural tube defects (alpha-fetoprotein testing not required) (NICE, 2008)

Screening for Down syndrome

Screening for Down syndrome should be performed by the end of the first trimester (13 weeks 6 days) but provision should be made for later screening (up to 20 weeks 0 days) for women booking later in pregnancy (NICE, 2008).

If a pregnant woman receives a screen-positive result for Down syndrome, she should have rapid access to counselling by trained staff (NICE, 2008).

Further reading

NICE, 2008, updated March 2016. Antenatal care for uncomplicated pregnancies. Clinical guideline 62. https://www.nice.org.uk/guidance/cg62.

Antepartum haemorrhage

Antepartum haemorrhage (APH) is bleeding from the genital tract after the 24th week of gestation and before the onset of labour.

Effect on the fetus

Fetal mortality and morbidity are increased as a result of severe vaginal bleeding in pregnancy. Stillbirth or neonatal death may occur. Premature placental separation and consequent hypoxia may result in severe neurological damage to the baby.

Effect on the mother

If bleeding is severe, it may be accompanied by shock and disseminated intravascular coagulation. The mother may die or be left with permanent ill-health.

Types of APH

+ Bleeding from local lesions of the genital tract (incidental causes)
+ Placental separation due to placenta praevia or placental abruption
See also Placenta.

Further reading

National Institute for Health and Care Excellence, 2014. Intrapartum care for healthy women and babies. Clinical guideline 190. https://www.nice.org.uk/guidance/cg190/chapter/Recommendations.
Royal College of Obstetricians and Gynaecologists, 2011. Antepartum haemorrhage. Green-top guideline no. 63. https://www.rcog.org.uk/globalassets/documents/guidelines/gtg_63.pdf.

Anticoagulation therapy

Required most commonly for patients at high risk of thromboembolism (blockage of a blood vessel by a clot or thrombus formed elsewhere in the blood system and carried in the circulation).

Venous thromboembolism (VTE) remains one of the main direct causes of maternal death. Better recognition of women at risk and more widespread use of thromboprophylaxis have led to a significant decline in such deaths.

VTE can occur at any time during pregnancy but women are at highest risk during the puerperium. All women should undergo a documented assessment of risk factors for VTE in early pregnancy or pre-pregnancy. Women with four or more risk factors should be considered for prophylactic low molecular weight heparin (LMWH) throughout the antenatal period. Aspirin is not recommended for thromboprophylaxis in obstetric patients. In clinically suspected deep vein thrombosis or pulmonary embolism, treatment with LMWH should be commenced immediately, unless treatment is strongly contraindicated.

In pregnancy, early activation of the clotting system may contribute to later pathology of preeclampsia. As a result, the use of anticoagulant or antiplatelet agents has been considered for the prevention of preeclampsia and fetal growth restriction. The World Health Organization (WHO) recommends low-dose aspirin (75 mg) *only* for women at high risk of developing the condition but evidence is limited.

> **Further reading**
>
> European Society of Cardiology. Guidelines for the management of cardiovascular diseases during pregnancy. How to manage anticoagulation in pregnant women. https://www.escardio.org/static_file/Escardio/Guidelines/publications/PREGN%20 Guidelines-Pregnancy-FT.pdf.
>
> Royal College of Obstetricians and Gynaecologists, 2015. Reducing the risk of venous thromboembolism during pregnancy and the puerperium. Green-top guideline no. 37a. https://www.rcog.org.uk/globalassets/documents/guidelines/gtg-37a.pdf.
>
> Royal College of Obstetricians and Gynaecologists, 2015. Thromboembolic disease in pregnancy and the puerperium: acute management. Green-top guideline no. 37b. https://www.rcog.org.uk/globalassets/documents/guidelines/gtg-37b.pdf.
>
> WHO, 2011. WHO recommendations for prevention and treatment of pre-eclampsia and eclampsia. http://www.ncbi.nlm.nih.gov/books/NBK140560/.

Anxiety See Perinatal mental health.

Apgar score

The Apgar score (Table 1) was developed in 1952 by Virginia Apgar as a means to quickly assess the health of newborn baby, particularly in the

Table 1 The Apgar score

Sign	Score[a]		
	0	1	2
Heart rate (beats/min)	Absent	<100	>100
Respiratory effort	Absent	Slow, irregular	Good or crying
Muscle tone	Limp	Some flexion of limbs	Active
Reflex response to stimuli	None	Minimal grimace	Cough or sneeze
Colour[b]	Blue, pale	Body pink, extremities blue	Completely pink

[a] Score is assessed at 1 and 5 minutes. Seek medical aid if total score is <7.
[b] 'Apgar minus colour' score omits fifth sign. Medical aid should be sought if total score is <6.

context of the effects of obstetric anaesthesia. It comprises evaluation of five criteria on a scale from 0 to 2, then summing the values, resulting in a score ranging from 0 to 10.

The criteria can be remembered with this mnemonic:

appearance
pulse (heart rate)
grimace (response to stimuli)
activity
respiration

Assessments should be performed at 1 and 5 minutes, for the further management of resuscitation (if required) (1 minute) and response to resuscitation (5 minutes). The higher the score, the better the outcome for the baby.

Further reading

National Institute for Health and Care Excellence, 2014. Intrapartum care for healthy women and babies. Clinical guideline 190. https://www.nice.org.uk/guidance/cg190/chapter/ Recommendations.

Arrhythmias, cardiac

An abnormal heart rhythm—rapid, slow and/or irregular—that is caused by disturbance in the heart's electrical conduction system.

Symptoms include: palpitations, breathlessness, light-headedness, dizziness or blackout, chest pain, angina. Rarely, some types of arrhythmia cause sudden death.

Arrhythmias in pregnancy are common and may cause concern for the wellbeing of both the mother and the fetus. For some women, the arrhythmia may be a recurrence of a previously diagnosed condition, or the first presentation in a woman with known structural heart disease. In most cases there is no previous history of heart disease.

The majority of arrhythmias in pregnancy are benign and advice and reassurance is generally all that is needed. In other cases, careful treatment with antiarrhythmic drugs will ensure a safe outcome for both the woman and the baby. In women with known structural heart disease, arrhythmia is a predictor of a cardiac event during pregnancy or labour (Adamson and Nelson-Piercy, 2007).

The heartbeat

- Adults: normal heart rate (sinus rhythm) is 60–100 beats/min at rest.
- Sinus bradycardia is a regular but slow heartbeat (<60 beats/min).

- Sinus tachycardia is a regular but fast heartbeat (>100 beats/min).
- Ectopic beats are extra heartbeats, common and usually normal. They can also manifest as skipped beats.
- Palpitations are an unpleasant awareness of the heartbeat—often described as 'thumping in the chest'—and can be quite normal.

Types of arrhythmia

- Atrial fibrillation: common; the atrial muscles flicker and the ventricles contract irregularly.
- Ventricular fibrillation: whole heart stops beating properly and just flutters; fatal unless heart is restarted with cardioversion (using a defibrillator).
- Atrial tachycardia and ventricular tachycardia: need urgent medical treatment.
- Heart block: an abnormally slow beat caused by the heart's electrical impulses not reaching the ventricles properly.

See also Cardiac disease in pregnancy.

Further reading

Adamson, D., Nelson-Piercy, C., 2007. Managing palpitations and arrhythmias during pregnancy. Heart 93 (12), 1630–1636. http://www.ncbi.nlm.nih.gov/pmc/articles/PMC2095764/.

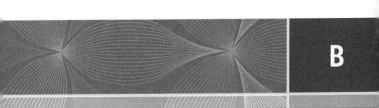

B

Bandl ring

An exaggerated retraction ring seen as an oblique ridge above the symphysis pubis between the upper and lower uterine segments—a sign of advanced, obstructed labour. This sign denotes a marked difference in thickness between the tonically retracted upper uterine segment and thinner lower segment, which is at risk of rupture. If allowed to persist, obstructed labour poses a high mortality risk to the fetus, the mother or both. By good antenatal care and close observation in early labour, the causes of obstructed labour can be recognized and treatment initiated before obstruction occurs.

Further reading

Macdonald, S., Magill-Cuerden, J. (Eds), 2011. Mayes' Midwifery, forteenth ed. Baillière Tindall, Elsevier, London.

World Health Organization. Managing prolonged and obstructed labour. Midwifery education module 3. http://www.who.int/maternal_child_adolescent/documents/3_9241546662/en/.

Bishop score

Rating system (Table 2) to assess the suitability of the cervix for induction of labour.

Table 2 Modified bishop preinduction pelvic scoring system[a]

Inducibility features[b]	0	1	2	3
Dilatation of cervix (cm)	<1	1–2	2–4	>4
Consistency of cervix	Firm	Firm	Medium	Soft
Cervical canal length (cm)	>4	2–4	1–2	<1
Position of cervix	Posterior	Mid	Anterior	–
Position of presenting part (cm above or below ischial spine)	–3	–2	–1	+1, +2

[a]A score of 8 or more denotes a ripe cervix that is amenable to induction of labour.
[b]Note: a vaginal examination to assess the cervix is a subjective examination and may be subject to interobserver variation.

Blood pressure

Blood pressure (BP) is taken to ascertain normality and provide a baseline reading for comparison throughout pregnancy.

- Systolic BP may be falsely elevated if the woman is nervous or anxious; a full bladder can cause an increase in BP.
- The woman should be seated or resting in a lateral position on the couch when BP is taken.
- A systolic BP of 140 mmHg or diastolic pressure of 90 mmHg at booking is indicative of hypertension and will need careful monitoring throughout pregnancy.

Sphygmomanometers should be calibrated for use in pregnancy and regularly maintained. The correct size cuff for the woman should be used—BP can be overestimated as a result of using a cuff of inadequate size relative to the arm circumference. Two cuffs should be available with inflation bladders of 35 cm for normal use and 42 cm for large arms. BP should be recorded as accurately as possible to the nearest 2 mmHg.

BP over 140/90 mmHg when accompanied by proteinuria (>1+ on dipstick or >0.3 g/L in a clean catch specimen) is suspicious for preeclampsia. BP over 140/90 mmHg in the absence of proteinuria but accompanied by headache, blurred vision, abdominal/epigastric pain or altered biochemistry may also indicate preeclampsia.

Hypertension

May be chronic and preexisting prior to pregnancy or gestational, developing during pregnancy (pregnancy induced hypertension) with or without other signs of preeclampsia.

Further reading

American Congress of Obstetricians and Gynecologists, 2014.
    Preeclampsia and high blood pressure during pregnancy.
    Information for patients. http://www.acog.org/Patients/FAQs/
    Preeclampsia-and-High-Blood-Pressure-During-Pregnancy.
National Institute of Health and Care Excellence, 2010, updated 2011.
    Hypertension in pregnancy: diagnosis and management. Clinical
    guideline 107. https://www.nice.org.uk/guidance/cg107.

Body mass index (BMI)

An indirect measure of body fat. Identifies possible weight problems for adults, and allows individuals to compare their weight status to that of the general population. BMI = weight (kg)/height (m)^2.

Interpretation of BMI in adults

- Overweight: BMI of 25–29.9 kg/m^2
- Obesity I: BMI of 30–34.9 kg/m^2
- Obesity II: BMI of 35–39.9 kg/m^2
- Obesity III: BMI of 40 kg/m^2 or more

BMI takes no account of fat distribution or body composition; for example, a highly trained athlete may have a high BMI because of increased muscularity rather than increased body fat.

Further reading

National Institute of Health and Care Excellence (NICE), 2010. Weight management before, during and after pregnancy. Public health guideline 27. https://www.nice.org.uk/guidance/ph27.

NICE, 2014. Obesity: identification, assessment and management. Clinical guideline 189. https://www.nice.org.uk/guidance/cg189.

NHS Choices, 2015. Overweight and pregnant. http://www.nhs.uk/conditions/pregnancy-and-baby/pages/overweight-pregnant.aspx.

Royal College of Obstetricians and Gynaecologists (RCOG), 2010. Management of women with obesity in pregnancy. https://www.rcog.org.uk/en/guidelines-research-services/guidelines/management-of-women-with-obesity-in-pregnancy/.

RCOG, 2011. Why your weight matters during pregnancy and after birth. https://www.rcog.org.uk/en/patients/patient-leaflets/why-your-weight-matters-during-pregnancy-and-after-birth/.

Booking interview

The purpose of the booking[1] visit or initial antenatal assessment is to:

+ introduce the woman to the maternity service
+ share information in order to discuss, plan and implement care for the duration of the pregnancy, the birth and postnatally

The earlier first contact is made with the midwife, the more appropriate and valuable the advice given relating to nutrition and care of the developing fetal organs. Medical conditions, infections, smoking, alcohol and drug taking may all have a profound and detrimental effect on the fetus at this time.

Among the topics to be covered are:

+ social history
+ general health
+ menstrual history
+ obstetric history
+ medical history
+ family history

---

[1]The term 'booking' interview, although still used in practice, was originally used to describe the pregnant woman 'booking' with her choice of maternity provider and 'booking' in for her birth. This reflects the funding stream rather than the care required.

In addition to general observations, the midwife should undertake a physical examination, blood pressure, urinalysis and blood tests. (See Antenatal care, Antenatal examination and Antenatal screening.)

Bradycardia

Bradycardia is an abnormally slow heart rate, defined as under 60 beats per minute in adults. Pathological bradycardia in pregnant women is rare. Some women who have physiological bradycardia may, in the second trimester, feel symptomatic as their blood pressure drops due to a reduction in systemic resistance; however, treatment is rarely required. Rarely, symptomatic bradycardia has been attributed to supine hypotensive syndrome of pregnancy, which is a result of compression of the inferior vena cava by the gravid uterus and responds to maternal changing of position (Adamson and Nelson-Piercy, 2007).

Bradycardia may also be caused by opioids (e.g. morphine, diamorphine, pethidine) administered during labour. Opioids reduce the heart rate by direct action on the cardiovascular centres in the medulla, by decreasing the activity of the sympathetic nervous system and by reducing anxiety. In labour this may contribute to a fall in blood pressure and reduction in placental perfusion. The subsequent depression of the fetal heart rate may be interpreted as fetal distress, prompting medical intervention. Some fetal bradycardia on administration of opioid analgesia by any route is normal, but a significant change in fetal heart rate is an indication of fetal compromise.

Further reading

Adamson, D., Nelson-Piercy, C., 2007. Managing palpitations and arrhythmias during pregnancy. Heart 93, 1630–1636. http://heart.bmj.com/content/93/12/1630.

Breastfeeding

The World Health Organization strongly recommends exclusive breastfeeding for the first 6 months of life. Most women are able to breastfeed.

Breastfeeding should be promoted in a sensitive manner, and information given about the benefits to both mother and baby, evidence for which is well established, as it is for the risks of not breastfeeding (United Nations Children's Fund [UNICEF]).

Babies who breastfeed are at lower risk of:

+ gastroenteritis
+ respiratory infections and asthma

+ sudden infant death syndrome
+ obesity
+ type 1 and type 2 diabetes
+ allergies (e.g. lactose intolerance)

Benefits to mothers

+ The longer mothers breastfeed, the greater their protection against breast and ovarian cancer, and hip fractures in later life.
+ Recent evidence has demonstrated an association between prolonged breastfeeding and postmenopausal risk factors for cardiovascular disease.
+ The World Cancer Research Fund includes breastfeeding as one of 10 recommendations to reduce the risk of some cancers.

These illnesses represent the greatest threats to women's health across all ages.

Evidence also suggests that breastfeeding has a positive impact on mother–baby relationships, conducive to the baby's health and emotional, social and physical development.

In the UK, the initial breastfeeding rate is 81%, according to the 5-yearly Infant Feeding Survey, 2010. (The survey scheduled for 2015 was cancelled.) Key findings of the survey were:

+ The initial breastfeeding rate increased from 76% in 2005 to 81% in 2010. This includes all babies who were put to the breast at all, even if this was on one occasion only, and also includes giving expressed breastmilk.
+ The highest incidences of breastfeeding were found among mothers aged 30 or over (87%), those from minority ethnic groups (97% for Chinese mothers or other ethnic group, 96% for black and 95% for Asian mothers), those who left education aged over 18 years (91%), those in managerial and professional occupations (90%) and those living in the least deprived areas (89%).
+ The prevalence of breastfeeding fell from 81% at birth to 69% at 1 week, and to 55% at 6 weeks. At 6 months, just over a third of mothers (34%) were still breastfeeding.
+ Mothers continued to breastfeed for longer in 2010 than was the case in 2005. The gap in breastfeeding levels at birth between 2005 and 2010 was five percentage points (76% in 2005 compared with 81% in 2010) and by 6 months the gap became nine percentage points (25% in 2005 compared to 34% in 2010). This suggests that policy developments to improve support and information provided to mothers to encourage them to continue breastfeeding may have had an impact.
+ Across the UK, 69% of mothers were exclusively breastfeeding at birth in 2010. At 1 week, less than half of all mothers (46%) were exclusively

breastfeeding, while this had fallen to around a quarter (23%) by 6 weeks. By 6 months, levels of exclusive breastfeeding had decreased to 1%, indicating that very few mothers were following the UK health departments' recommendation that babies should be exclusively breastfed until around the age of 6 months.

• There has been an increase in the prevalence of exclusive breastfeeding at birth (from 65% in 2005 to 69% in 2010), but there has been little change thereafter up until 6 weeks. However, the opt-out rate in later months was lower in 2010 than 2005. For example, at 3 months, 17% of mothers were still breastfeeding exclusively (up from 13% in 2005) and at 4 months, 12% were still breastfeeding exclusively (up from 7% in 2005).

Breastfeeding rates in the US are similar to those in the UK (Health and Social Care Information Centre [HSCIC], 2012).

The UNICEF UK Baby Friendly Initiative standards recommend healthcare professionals to:

1. Support pregnant women to recognize the importance of breastfeeding and early relationships for the health and well-being of their baby.
2. Support all mothers and babies to initiate a close relationship and feeding soon after birth.
3. Enable mothers to get breastfeeding off to a good start.
4. Support mothers to make informed decisions regarding the introduction of food or fluids other than breastmilk.
5. Support parents to have a close and loving relationship with their baby.

Early feeding contributes to the success of breastfeeding. The first feed should be supervised by the midwife. It should proceed without pain and baby should be allowed to terminate the feed spontaneously.

Certain preexisting conditions, most notably HIV, are a contraindication to breastfeeding due to the risk of vertical transmission of the infection from the mother to the baby.

See also Lactation.

Further reading/resources

Bartick, M., Reinhold, A., 2010. The burden of suboptimal breastfeeding in the United States: a pediatric cost analysis. Pediatrics 125 (5), e1048–e1056. http://www.ncbi.nlm.nih.gov/pubmed/20368314.

Continued

Further reading/resources—cont'd

HSCIC, 2012. Infant Feeding Survey—UK, 2010. http://content.digital.
nhs.uk/catalogue/PUB08694/Infant-Feeding-Survey-2010-
Consolidated-Report.pdf.

Patient. Infant feeding (professional reference). http://patient.info/
doctor/infant-feeding.

UNICEF. Health benefits of breastfeeding. https://www.unicef.org.uk/
babyfriendly/what-is-baby-friendly/the-benefits-of-breastfeeding/.

UNICEF UK, 2012. Guide to the Baby Friendly Initiative standards.
https://www.unicef.org.uk/babyfriendly/baby-friendly-resources/
guidance-for-health-professionals/implementing-the-baby-friendly-
standards/guide-to-the-baby-friendly-initiative-standards/.

Information/further reading for patients

BFN—The Breastfeeding Network. http://www.breastfeedingnetwork.
org.uk.

La Leche League GB. http://www.laleche.org.uk.

National Childbirth Trust (NCT). http://www.nct.org.uk.

NHS Choices. Pregnancy and baby guide. http://www.nhs.uk/
Conditions/pregnancy-and-baby/pages/pregnancy-and-baby-care
.aspx.

Payne, J., 2016. Breast feeding (information for patients).
http://patient.info/health/breast-feeding-leaflet.

Breastmilk

Human milk varies in its composition. The most dramatic change in the composition of milk occurs during the course of a feed. At the beginning of the feed the baby receives a high volume of relatively low-fat milk, but as the feed progresses, the volume decreases but the proportion of fat increases. The baby's ability to obtain this fat-rich milk is not determined by the length of the feed but by the quality of the attachment to the breast.

It is the fat and not the protein in human milk that has particular significance.

+ In human milk, 98% of the lipid is in the form of triglycerides.
+ Over 100 fatty acids have so far been identified.
+ Fat provides the baby with more than 50% of his/her calorific requirements.

Human milk also provides carbohydrate, in the form of lactose; protein; vitamins A, D, E, K and C; minerals and trace elements, including iron, zinc and calcium; antiinfective factors including leucocytes, especially in the first 10 days of life when there are more white cells per millilitre in breast milk than in blood; immunoglobulins; lysozyme; lactoferrin; bifidus factor and hormones; and growth factors.

Further reading

Ballard, O., Morrow, A., 2013. Human milk composition: nutrients and bioactive factors. Pediatr Clin North Am 60 (1), 49–74. https://www.ncbi.nlm.nih.gov/pmc/articles/PMC3586783/.
Infant Nutrition Council (Australia & New Zealand). Breastmilk information. http://www.infantnutritioncouncil.com/resources/breastmilk-information/.

Breech presentation

Breech is the most commonly encountered malpresentation. Its incidence decreases with gestational age: at 32 weeks' gestation approximately 20% of fetuses present with breech but the incidence decreases to 3%–4% at term.

The four types of breech position are:
+ breech with extended legs (frank breech) (Fig. 2)
+ complete breech (Fig. 3)
+ footling breech (Fig. 4)
+ knee presentation (Fig. 5)

Often no cause is identified, but the following factors favour breech presentation:
+ extended legs
+ preterm labour
+ multiple pregnancy

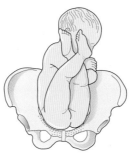

Fig. 2 Breech with extended legs (frank breech).

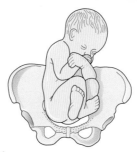

Fig. 3 **Complete breech.**

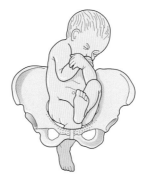

Fig. 4 **Footling breech.**

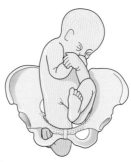

Fig. 5 **Knee presentation.**

- polyhydramnios
- hydrocephaly
- uterine abnormalities
- placenta praevia

Breech presentation can be diagnosed antenatally by abdominal palpation, during auscultation (the fetal heart is auscultated higher) or with ultrasound.

During labour it is diagnosed by abdominal examination, vaginal examination (where the breech is felt as soft and irregular with no sutures palpable; the anus may be felt and fresh meconium on the examining finger is usually diagnostic). If the legs are extended, the external genitalia are very evident; and a foot may be differentiated from a hand.

Careful assessment should be made at the start of labour, and anticipated labour management should be reviewed. A consultant obstetrician should be informed.

Types of vaginal breech birth

- Spontaneous (little or no assistance from the attendant)
- Assisted (the buttocks are born spontaneously but some assistance is necessary for delivery of extended legs or arms and the head)
- Breech extraction (manipulative delivery carried out by an obstetrician to hasten delivery in an emergency situation such as fetal compromise)

In the first stage of labour, meconium-stained liquor is sometimes found due to compression of the fetal abdomen, and is not always a sign of fetal compromise. A vaginal examination should be performed to exclude cord prolapse. In a hospital setting, the obstetrician should be informed at the onset of second stage, and a paediatrician should be present for the birth. Full dilatation of the cervix should be confirmed before the woman starts to push. Active pushing is commenced when the buttocks are distending the vulva. Failure of the breech to descend onto the perineum despite good contractions may indicate the need for caesarean section.

The buttocks should be born spontaneously. If the legs are flexed, the feet disengage at the vulva and the baby is born as far as the umbilicus. If the legs are extended, intervention is usually needed to ease their delivery, by placing a finger in the popliteal fossa and gently flexing the knee. The midwife should feel for the elbows, which are usually on the chest. If so, they will escape at the next contraction. If the arms are not felt, they are extended. Since the arms and head cannot be delivered together, interventions such as the Løvset manoeuvre may need to be performed (see Løvset manoeuvre).

There are three methods of delivering the head—the Burns–Marshall method, the Mauriceau–Smellie–Veit manoeuvre (see individual entries) and forceps delivery. Most breech births are performed by an obstetrician who will apply forceps to the after-coming head to achieve a controlled delivery.

Burns–Marshall method

A method of breech delivery when the head is flexed involving traction to prevent the neck from bending backwards and being fractured (see also Breech presentation).

The baby's feet are grasped in the nondominant hand, and sufficient traction applied to prevent the neck from bending backwards and being fractured. The suboccipital region and not the neck should pivot under the apex of the pubic arch to prevent the spinal cord from being crushed. The feet are taken through an arc of 180 degrees until the mouth and nose are free at the vulva. The right (or dominant) hand may guard the perineum to prevent sudden escape of the head. The mother should be asked to take deliberate, regular breaths that allow the vault of the skull to escape gradually.

Further reading

Royal College of Obstetricians and Gynaecologists, 2006. Management of breech presentation. Guideline 20. https://www.rcog.org.uk/globalassets/documents/gtg-no-20b-breech-presentation.pdf.

C

Caesarean section

An operative procedure carried out under anaesthesia whereby the fetus, placenta and membranes are delivered through an incision in the abdominal wall and the uterus.

Emergency caesarean section (C section) is carried out when adverse conditions develop during pregnancy or labour. Examples of indications for emergency C section include:

- antepartum haemorrhage
- cord prolapse
- uterine rupture
- cephalopelvic disproportion diagnosed in labour
- fulminating preeclampsia, eclampsia
- fetal compromise if birth is not imminent

Elective C section is so termed when the decision to carry out the procedure has been taken during pregnancy, before labour has commenced. Indications include:

Definite
- Cephalopelvic disproportion
- Major degree of placenta praevia
- High-order multiple pregnancy

Possible
- Breech presentation
- Moderate to severe preeclampsia
- Medical condition that warrants the exclusion of maternal effort
- Diabetes mellitus
- Intrauterine growth restriction
- Certain fetal abnormalities (e.g. hydrocephalus)
- Antepartum haemorrhage

Regional anaesthesia remains the safer option but general anaesthesia is sometimes required.
- Regional anaesthesia is incompatible with maternal coagulation disorders.
- General anaesthesia can be administered more rapidly.
- Maternal preference may be for general anaesthesia.

Complications can include infection and thromboembolic disorders (see also Vaginal birth after caesarean section).

Further reading

National Institute of Health and Care Excellence, 2011, updated 2012. Caesarean section. Clinical guideline 132. https://www.nice.org .uk/guidance/cg132.

Caput succedaneum (Fig. 6)

Caput succedaneum is the swelling of the scalp in a newborn. It is most often brought on by pressure exerted from the uterus or vaginal wall during a vertex (head first) delivery, where progress is slow or temporarily obstructed, normally due to the position or flexion of the head. It is a soft,

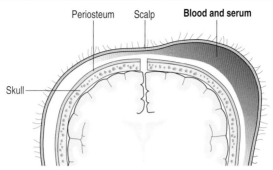

Fig. 6 Caput succedaneum.

puffy swelling on the scalp, with possible bruising or change of colour. A caput succedaneum is more likely to form during a long or hard delivery and is more common after the membranes have broken, as the amniotic fluid no longer provides a cushion for the baby's head. It is most often seen on the portion of the head that presented first.

Features of caput succedaneum

* Is present at birth
* Does not usually enlarge
* Can 'pit' on pressure
* Can cross a suture line
* Involves oedema that may move to the dependent area of the scalp
* Usually resolves by 36 hours of life
* Has no long-term consequences

Ventouse extraction may increase the chance of a 'false' caput succedaneum, an oedematous deformity also known as a chignon.

Further reading

Patient, 2015. Birth injuries to the baby. (Professional reference.)
    http://patient.info/doctor/birth-injuries-to-the-baby.

Cardiac disease in pregnancy

In most pregnancies, heart disease is diagnosed before pregnancy. There is, however, a small but significant group of women who will present at an antenatal clinic with an undiagnosed heart condition. Cardiac disease takes a variety of forms. Those more likely to be seen in pregnancy are rheumatic heart disease and congenital heart disease.

Common congenital heart defects in pregnancy

+ Atrial septal defect
+ Ventricular septal defect
+ Patent ductus arteriosus
+ Pulmonary stenosis
+ Aortic stenosis
+ Tetralogy of Fallot
+ Eisenmenger syndrome
+ Marfan syndrome

Acquired heart conditions

+ Aortic dissection (acute)
+ Rheumatic heart disease
+ Ischaemic heart disease
+ Endocarditis
+ Peripartum cardiomyopathy

Changes in cardiovascular dynamics during pregnancy

In normal pregnancy the haemodynamic profile alters in order to meet the increasing demands of the growing fetoplacental unit. Although this increases the workload of the heart quite significantly, normal, healthy pregnant women are able to adjust to these physiological changes easily. In women with coexisting heart disease, however, the added workload can precipitate complications. The haemodynamic changes commence early in pregnancy and gradually reach their maximum effect between 28 and 32 weeks.

During labour there is a significant increase in cardiac output as a result of uterine contractions.

In the 12–24 hours following birth there is further alteration with the shift of blood (approximately 1 L) from the uterine to the systemic circulation.

Diagnosis

The recognition of heart disease in pregnancy may be difficult, as many of the symptoms of normal pregnancy resemble those of heart disease.

Common signs and symptoms of cardiac compromise in pregnancy

+ Fatigue
+ Shortness of breath (dyspnoea)

- Difficulty in breathing unless upright (orthopnoea)
- Palpitations
- Bounding/collapsing pulse
- Chest pain
- Development of peripheral oedema
- Distended jugular veins
- Progressive limitation of physical activity

Laboratory tests can assist with the diagnosis of cardiac disease and help with the assessment of current functional capacity. Tests include:

- full blood count
- electrocardiography (ECG)
- chest radiograph to assess cardiac size and outline, pulmonary vasculature and lung fields
- clotting studies
- echocardiography

Risks to mother and fetus

The majority of pregnancies complicated by maternal heart disease can be expected to have a favourable outcome for both mother and fetus. The risk for morbidity and mortality depends on:

- the nature of the cardiac lesion,
- its effect on the functional capacity of the heart,

- the development of pregnancy-related complications such as hypertensive disorders of pregnancy, infection, thrombosis and haemorrhage.

Preconception care

Women with known heart disease should seek advice from a cardiologist and an obstetrician before becoming pregnant, so that the risks of the condition can be discussed.

Antenatal care

The symptoms of normal pregnancy, together with the haemodynamic changes, can mimic the signs and symptoms of heart disease. Maternal investigations should be carried out prior to and at the onset of pregnancy in order to gain baseline referral points.

Management

All pregnant women with heart disease should be managed in obstetric units via a multidisciplinary approach involving midwives, obstetricians, cardiologists and anaesthetists. The aim is to maintain a steady haemodynamic state and prevent complications, as well as promote physical and psychological wellbeing. Visits to a joint clinic run by a cardiologist and obstetrician are usually made every 2 weeks until 30 weeks' gestation and weekly thereafter until birth. At each visit, functional grading is made according to the New York Heart Association classification and the severity of the heart lesion is assessed by clinical examination. Evaluation of fetal wellbeing will include:

- ultrasound examination to confirm gestational age and congenital abnormality,
- assessment of fetal growth and amniotic fluid volume, both clinically and by ultrasound,
- monitoring of the fetal heart rate by cardiotocography,
- measurement of fetal and maternal placental blood flow indices by Doppler ultrasonography.

Intrapartum care
The first stage of labour
Vaginal birth is preferred unless there is an obstetric indication for caesarean section. Optimal management involves monitoring the maternal condition closely. This will include the measurement of:

- temperature
- pulse
- respiration
- blood pressure
- urine output

Pulse oximetry, insertion of a central venous pressure catheter and ECG monitoring may be utilized.

Fluid balance
Women with significant heart disease require care to be taken concerning fluid balance in labour. Indiscriminate use of intravenous crystalloid fluids will lead to an increase in circulating blood volume, which women with heart disease will find difficult to cope with and they may easily develop pulmonary oedema.

Pain relief
It is important to consult a doctor before administering any form of pain-relieving drug to a woman with a heart condition. In the majority, an epidural would be the analgesia of choice.

Positioning
Cardiac output is influenced by the position of the labouring woman. It is preferable for an upright or left lateral position to be adopted.

Preterm labour

If a woman with heart disease should go into labour prematurely, then beta-sympathomimetic drugs are contraindicated.

Induction

The least stressful labour for a woman with cardiac disease will be spontaneous in onset; induction is considered safe only if the benefits outweigh the disadvantages.

The second stage of labour

This should be short without undue exertion on the part of the mother. The midwife should encourage the woman to breathe normally and follow her natural desire to push, giving several short pushes during each contraction.

Forceps or ventouse may be used to shorten the second stage if the maternal condition deteriorates.

Care should be taken when the woman is in the lithotomy position, as this produces a sudden increase in venous return to the heart, which may result in heart failure.

The third stage of labour

This is usually actively managed owing to the increased risk of postpartum haemorrhage (PPH). Oxytocin is the drug of choice but its use in the prevention of PPH must be balanced against the risk of oxytocin-induced hypotension and tachycardia in women with cardiovascular compromise.

Ergot-containing preparations such as ergometrine are contraindicated.

Postnatal care

During the first 48 hours following birth the heart must cope with the extra blood from the uterine circulation. Close observation should identify early signs of infection, thrombosis or pulmonary oedema.

Breastfeeding is not contraindicated.

Discharge planning is particularly important for women with heart disease. The woman and her partner will need to discuss the implications of a future pregnancy with the cardiologist and obstetrician.

Cardiotocography (Fig. 7)

Measurement of the fetal heart rate can be used to assess uterine contractions, although this should not completely replace palpation of contractions by the midwives. The aim of cardiotocography (CTG) is to identify changes

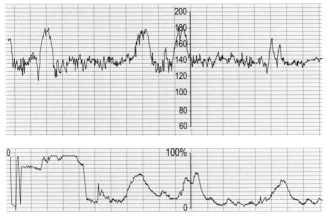

Fig. 7 Normal cardiotocograph with reassuring features (i.e., baseline variability, presence of accelerations and no decelerations).

to the fetal heart rate that may be indicative of a developing fetal compromise.

The cardiotocograph (Table 3, overleaf) provides information on:

* the baseline fetal heart rate
* baseline variability
* accelerations from the base rate
* decelerations from the base rate
* uterine activity

Women with a low-risk pregnancy should have intermittent auscultation with a Pinard stethoscope or hand-held Doppler device. There is no evidence to support CTG on admission. However, for women with a higher risk pregnancy, electronic fetal monitoring is appropriate.

The use of CTG may limit the choice of position for the woman in labour, although, increasingly, equipment to enable telemetry can help to minimize restrictions.

Further reading

National Institute for Health and Care Excellence, 2014. Intrapartum care for healthy women and babies. Clinical guideline 190. https://www.nice.org.uk/guidance/cg190.

NHS Litigation Authority, 2010. Maternity claims. Information sheet 7. CTG interpretation. http://www.nhsla.com/safety/Documents/CTG%20Interpretation%20-%207.pdf.

Continued

Table 3 Fetal heart rate assessment

CTG classification	
Normal	A CTG where all four features fall into the reassuring category
Suspicious	A CTG where features fall into one of the nonreassuring categories and the remaining features are reassuring
Pathological	A CTG where features fall into two or more nonreassuring categories or one or more abnormal categories

Fetal heart rate features classification

	Baseline (beats/min)	Variability (beats/min)	Decelerations	Accelerations
Reassuring	100–160 (110 may still be used in practice)	≥5	None	Present
Nonreassuring	100–109 161–180	≤5 for ≥40 min but <90 min	Early decelerations Variable decelerations Single prolonged deceleration up to 3 min	The absence of accelerations with an otherwise normal CTG is of uncertain significance
Abnormal	<100 >180 Sinusoidal pattern for ≥10 min	<5 for ≥90 min	Atypical variable decelerations Late decelerations Single prolonged deceleration >3 min	

Further reading—cont'd

Royal College of Midwives, 2012. Evidence based guidelines for midwifery-led care in labour. Intermittent auscultation. https://www.rcm.org.uk/sites/default/files/Intermittent%20Auscultation%20(IA)_0.pdf.

Cephalhaematoma

Cephalhaematoma is an effusion of blood (haematoma, bruise) under the periosteum that covers the skull. It can occur during vaginal birth when there is friction between the fetal skull and the maternal pelvic bones, but is more commonly associated with instrumental delivery, especially ventouse extraction. It affects between 1 and 12 in 100 babies. More than one bone of the skull may be affected, causing multiple haematomas.

Unlike caput succedaneum, it is not necessarily apparent at birth but may appear after 12 hours. The swelling grows larger over subsequent days and can persist for weeks. The swelling:

+ is circumscribed and firm
+ does not pit on pressure
+ does not cross a suture
+ is fixed

No treatment is necessary and the swelling subsides when the blood is reabsorbed. Erythrocyte breakdown in the extravasated blood may result in hyperbilirubinemia (jaundice).

Chorioamnionitis

Also known as intraamniotic infection, chorioamnionitis is an inflammation of the membranes and chorion of the placenta due to a bacterial infection. It typically results from bacteria ascending into the uterus from the vagina and is associated with longer duration of membrane rupture and/or prolonged labour.

Signs and symptoms include:

+ maternal fever (intrapartum temperature >37.8°C)
+ significant maternal tachycardia (>120 beats/min)
+ fetal tachycardia (>160–180 beats/min)
+ purulent or foul-smelling amniotic fluid or vaginal discharge
+ uterine tenderness
+ maternal leukocytosis (total blood leukocyte count >15,000–18,000 cells/μL)

The presence of two or more of the above criteria indicate an increased risk of neonatal sepsis.

Further reading

Medscape, 2017. Chorioamnionitis. http://emedicine.medscape.com/article/973237-overview.

MSD Manual, 2014. Intra-Amniotic Infection (Chorioamnionitis). http://www.msdmanuals.com/en-gb/professional/gynecology-and-obstetrics/abnormalities-of-pregnancy/intra–amniotic-infection.

Coombs test

Coombs test is used to detect antibodies that can destroy red blood cells. There are two types of Coombs test, direct and indirect: the former looks directly at red blood cells, the latter looks at the plasma and is generally used to check compatibility of donor blood and the recipient. In the context of midwifery, it is used in prenatal testing of pregnant women to detect antibodies in order to prevent haemolytic disease of the newborn.

The direct Coombs test is performed after birth, using a sample of cord blood, to confirm rhesus type, ABO blood group, haemoglobin and serum bilirubin levels and the presence of maternal antibodies on fetal red blood cells. A negative test indicates an absence of antibodies or sensitization.

Conjoined twins

Extremely rare malformation of monozygotic twinning resulting from the incomplete division of the fertilized oocyte. Delivery has to be by caesarean section. Separation of the babies is sometimes possible and will depend on how they are joined and which internal organs are involved.

Constipation

A useful definition of constipation is 'the passage of hard stools less frequently than the patient's own normal pattern' (British National Formulary).

The Bristol stool form scale is a means of assessing intestinal transit time.

- Types 1 and 2 indicate constipation; will be passed infrequently.
- Types 3 and 4 indicate 'normal' ideal stools; should be passed once every 1–3 days, depending on individual normal bowel-emptying patterns.
- Types 5 to 7 suggest diarrhoea or urgency; passed very frequently.

The Bristol Stool Chart is available at https://www.hct.nhs.uk/media/1067/bristol-stool-chart.pdf.

Women may be more likely to experience constipation very early in pregnancy as a result of hormonal changes. Constipation is a common side effect of iron supplementation. Management involves increasing dietary fibre, exercise and drinking plenty of water. If dietary changes are insufficient to alleviate constipation, a laxative can be used. Those that are safe to use in pregnancy include lactulose and macrogols, which are not absorbed by the digestive tract. Stimulant laxatives such as senna may be unsuitable in later pregnancy because they are partially absorbed.

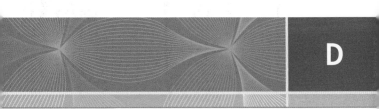

D

Depression

The most common mental health problem is a serious underdetected condition in which severe feelings of sadness, hopelessness and loss of interest in life interfere with daily life and can last for weeks or months. Depression can affect anyone, and it can occur in all age groups, including children and adolescents. Long-term medical conditions increase risk of major depression. A family history of depression also increases risk.

Clinical features of depression

- Symptoms of low mood: little interest (anhedonia), poor concentration, apathy/helplessness/hopelessness, tearfulness, pessimism
- Somatic symptoms: poor appetite, weight loss, insomnia, constipation, low libido
- Psychotic symptoms: hallucinations, delusions

Screening for depression

The National Institute for Health and Care Excellence (NICE) guidance advises screening high-risk groups, e.g., if past history of depression, significant physical illnesses causing disability and/or long-term conditions, using two questions concerning mood and interest:

1. During the past month have you often been bothered by feeling down, depressed or hopeless?

2. During the past month have you often been bothered by having little interest or pleasure in doing things?

A 'no' response to both questions makes depression highly unlikely. A 'yes' answer to either question is considered a positive test and the person should be:

+   first asked 'Is this something you feel you need or want help with?'
+   then reviewed by a practitioner competent in mental health assessment. Mixed anxiety/depression is common.

Postnatal depression

Postnatal depression is a nonpsychotic depressive illness of mild to moderate severity arising within 3 months of childbirth.

Main characteristics are:

+   Diurnal mood changes and sleep disturbance—waking early in the morning; the woman will feel most depressed and her symptoms will be worse at the start of the day
+   Impaired concentration, disturbed thought processes, indecisiveness and an inability to cope with everyday life
+   Emotional detachment and profound lowering of mood
+   Loss of ability to feel pleasure (anhedonia)
+   Feelings of guilt, incompetence and of being a 'bad' mother
+   In approximately one-third of women, distressing, intrusive obsessional thoughts
+   Commonly, extreme anxiety and even panic attacks
+   Impaired appetite and weight loss
+   In a small number, depressive psychosis, morbid, delusional thoughts and hallucinations

The Edinburgh Postnatal Depression Scale is a useful screening tool but can lead to 'false positives' and medicalization of low mood and situational distress; it should not replace clinical judgement.

Further reading/resources

MIND (merged with the Depression Alliance in 2016). Information and support. https://www.mind.org.uk/information-support/.

NICE, 2009, updated 2016. Depression. The treatment and management of depression in adults. Clinical guideline 90. https://www.nice.org.uk/guidance/cg90.

NICE, 2009. Depression in adults with a chronic physical health problem: recognition and management. Clinical guideline 91. http://www.nice.org.uk/CG91.

Further reading/resources—cont'd

Samaritans. http://www.samaritans.org or Tel.: 116 123 (UK/Republic of Ireland).

SIGN 114, 2010. Non-pharmaceutical management of depression. http://sign.ac.uk/guidelines/fulltext/114/index.html.

Disseminated intravascular coagulation

Disseminated intravascular coagulation (DIC) is a condition in which blood clots form throughout the body's small blood vessels, reducing or blocking blood flow through blood vessels leading to organ damage. In DIC, increased clotting uses up available platelets and clotting factors, which can lead to a serious bleeding risk.

Risk factors for DIC in pregnancy and/or labour include:

+ placental abruption
+ intrauterine fetal death, including delayed miscarriage
+ amniotic fluid embolism
+ intrauterine infection, including septic abortion
+ preeclampsia and eclampsia

DIC can cause life-threatening bleeding. Management involves replacement of platelets and clotting factors via frozen plasma and platelet concentrations, with subsequent transfusion of red blood cells.

Domestic abuse

One in *three* women experience domestic abuse or violence at some point in their lives. This may be physical, sexual, emotional, *financial* or psychological abuse. Thirty percent of this abuse starts in pregnancy and existing abuse may get worse during pregnancy or after giving birth.

Domestic abuse in pregnancy increases the risk of miscarriage, infection, premature birth and injury or death to the baby.

Women in abusive relationships are also more vulnerable to mental health problems including anxiety and postnatal depression.

When violence is suspected[1] the best way to confirm suspicion is by direct questioning, such as:

+ has someone been hurting you?
+ did somebody cause these injuries?
+ do you ever feel frightened of your partner or other people at home?

---

[1]Routine enquiry about domestic violence should only be carried out if appropriate education and training has been provided.

The woman may choose to deny being abused but awareness that help is available is useful. Fostering a safe, nurturing and private environment during antenatal visits, with the midwife expressing empathy and honesty, may provide the woman with an opportunity to seek help.

The midwife should understand the nature of domestic violence, be sensitive to clues that may suggest abuse and be aware of the impact of abuse on everyday life. Each maternity unit and midwifery group practice should have current details about domestic violence units and support groups for women.

Recent research (Donovan, 2016) confirms that physical assaults on pregnant women can directly affect a growing fetus, with a twofold increase in the risk of preterm birth and low birth weight.

Further reading/resources

Donovan, B.M., Spracklen, C.N., Schweizer, M.L., Ryckman, K.K., Saftlas, A.F., 2016. Intimate partner violence during pregnancy and the risk for adverse infant outcomes: a systematic review and meta-analysis. Br J Obstet Gynecol 123 (8), 1289–1299. http://onlinelibrary.wiley.com/doi/10.1111/1471-0528.13928/full.
National Domestic Violence Helpline. Tel.: +44-(0)808-2000-247.
Women's Aid. https://www.womensaid.org.uk.

Dystocia

Dystocia means literally 'difficult labour' and is associated with slowness or lack of progress. Possible causes include:

- contractions ineffective in dilating and effacing the cervix
- uncoordinated contractions where the two segments of the uterus fail to work in harmony
- contractions producing inadequate involuntary expulsion
- abnormalities of fetal presentation and position, the pelvis, the birth canal and congenital abnormalities
- full bladder, rectum or fibroids
  See also Shoulder dystocia

Eclampsia

Eclampsia, considered a complication of severe preeclampsia, is commonly defined as a new onset of seizures and/or unexplained coma during pregnancy or postpartum in a woman with signs or symptoms of preeclampsia, although it can develop independently of preeclampsia.

Eclampsia is rarely seen in developed countries. It has an incidence of 2.1 per 10,000 maternities in the UK. Eclampsia is associated with increased risks of maternal and perinatal morbidity and mortality. Significant maternal life-threatening complications as a result of eclampsia include:

+ pulmonary oedema
+ renal and hepatic failure
+ placental abruption and haemorrhage
+ disseminated intravascular coagulation
+ haemolysis, elevated liver enzymes, and low platelet count (HELLP) syndrome (see separate entry)
+ cerebral haemorrhage

Hypertension is not necessarily a precursor to the onset of eclampsia but will almost always be evident following a seizure.

The aims of immediate care are to preserve the mother's life: summon medical aid, clear and maintain the mother's airway, administer oxygen and prevent injury. Intravenous anticonvulsant and antihypertensive therapies will be administered according to protocol, and it is usual to expedite delivery of the baby, usually via caesarean section.

Further reading

National Institute for Health and Care Excellence (NICE), 2016. NICE pathways. Severe hypertension, severe pre-eclampsia and eclampsia in critical care. http://pathways.nice.org.uk/pathways/hypertension-in-pregnancy/severe-hypertension-severe-pre-eclampsia-and-eclampsia-in-critical-care.

NICE, 2015. Clinical Knowledge Summaries. Hypertension in pregnancy. http://cks.nice.org.uk/hypertension-in-pregnancy.

Ross, M., 2015, updated 2016. Eclampsia. Medscape. http://emedicine.medscape.com/article/253960-overview.

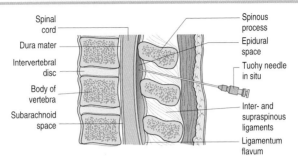

Fig. 8 Administration of epidural analgesia.

Epidural

Epidural or regional analgesia can provide effective pain relief during labour. Pain relief from an epidural is obtained by blocking the conduction of impulses along sensory nerves as they enter the spinal cord. The procedure is usually carried out by an experienced obstetric anaesthetist under strict aseptic conditions. A local anaesthetic is injected into the epidural space of the lumbar region, usually between vertebrae L1 and L2, or L2 and L3, or between L3 and L4 (Fig. 8). A continuous infusion of local anaesthetic (bupivacaine) and opioids (usually fentanyl) is administered via a syringe pump. In some instances, midwives top up the epidural block by giving a further dose as prescribed by the anaesthetist. The midwife is personally responsible for ensuring she is competent to carry out the procedure and should be aware of possible complications and their immediate treatment.

Complications may include:
+ dural puncture and consequent headache
+ total spinal block leading to respiratory arrest
+ local anaesthetic toxicity leading to cardiac arrest
+ fetal compromise (resulting from hypotension or local analgesic toxicity)
+ increased need for assisted vaginal birth
+ neurological sequelae (serious damage is extremely rare; weakness/ sensory loss is uncommon but soon resolves)
+ loss of bladder sensation

Further reading

National Institute for Health and Care Excellence, 2014. Intrapartum care for health women and babies. Clinical guideline 190. https://www.nice.org.uk/guidance/cg190/chapter/Recommendations.
Royal College of Anaesthetists Faculty of Pain Medicine, 2010. Best practice in the management of epidural analgesia in the hospital setting. https://www.aagbi.org/sites/default/files/epidural_analgesia_2011.pdf.

Entonox

Entonox is a 50 : 50 mixture of nitrous oxide and oxygen. It is an effective analgesic agent with rapid onset and offset characteristics. Its effects are predictable and reliable with minimal side effects. It is widely used, but its mechanism of action has not been fully explained.

In large obstetric units the gas is piped, but in the UK, smaller units and the community it is supplied in cylinders (blue with a blue and white shoulder). It is self-administered, but the woman needs to be adequately informed of the functioning of the apparatus. Optimal analgesia is obtained by closely applying the lips around the mouthpiece: the gases take effect within 20 seconds, so it is important that the woman uses it before a contraction. Maximum efficacy is achieved after 45–50 seconds, and, if correctly timed, this should coincide with the height of the contraction.

The use of scavenging equipment to extract expired gases is recommended for all birthing rooms.

Further reading

BOC 2015. Entonox®—the essential guide. http://www.bochealthcare.co.uk/internet.lh.lh.gbr/en/images/entonox_essential_guide_hlc401955_Sep10409_64836.pdf.

Episiotomy

Episiotomy (Fig. 9) is an incision through the perineal tissues to enlarge the vulval outlet during the birth. The rationale for its use depends on the need to minimize the risk of severe, spontaneous maternal trauma and to expedite the birth when there is evidence of fetal compromise. The woman needs to give consent prior to the procedure.

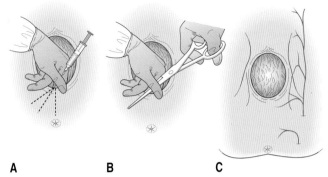

A   **B**   **C**

Fig. 9 (A) Infiltrating the perineum. (B) Performing an episiotomy. (C) Innervation of the vulval area and perineum.

- The perineum should be adequately anaesthetized prior to the incision (lidocaine 0.5% 10 mL or 1% 5 mL).
- The incision is made during a contraction when the tissues are stretched so that there is a clear view of the area and bleeding is less likely to be severe.
- Birth of the head should follow immediately and its advance must be controlled to avoid extension of the episiotomy.

There are two types of incision:

- Mediolateral: begins at the midpoint of the fourchette and is directed at a 45-degree angle to the midline towards a point midway between the ischial tuberosity and the anus.
- Median: a midline incision that follows the natural line of insertion of the perineal muscles. It is associated with reduced blood loss but a higher incidence of damage to the anal sphincter.

Further reading

Royal College of Midwives, 2012. Evidence based guidelines for midwifery-led care in labour. https://www.rcm.org.uk/sites/default/files/Care%20of%20the%20Perineum.pdf.

Ectopic pregnancy

An ectopic pregnancy is one where implantation occurs at a site other than the uterine cavity. Sites can include:

+ a fallopian (uterine) tube
+ an ovary
+ the cervix
+ the abdomen

Women require prompt, appropriate treatment for this life-threatening condition. Midwives need to consider the possibility of an ectopic pregnancy being responsible for unexplained abdominal pain and bleeding in early pregnancy.

Risk factors for ectopic pregnancy

Any of the alterations of the normal function of the uterine tube in transporting the gametes contributes to the risk of ectopic pregnancy.

+ Previous ectopic pregnancy
+ Previous tubal surgery
+ Emergency contraception in current pregnancy
+ Congenital abnormalities of the tube
+ Previous infection including chlamydia, gonorrhoea or pelvic inflammatory disease
+ Conception with intrauterine contraceptive device in situ
+ Assisted reproductive techniques
+ Smoking

Clinical presentation

Typical signs

+ Localized abdominal pain
+ Amenorrhoea
+ Vaginal bleeding or spotting

Atypical signs

+ Shoulder pain
+ Abdominal distension
+ Nausea, vomiting
+ Dizziness, fainting

Tubal pregnancy rarely remains asymptomatic beyond 8 weeks.

+ Pelvic pain can be severe.
+ Acute symptoms are the result of tubal rupture and relate to the degree of haemorrhage there has been.
+ Ultrasound enables an accurate diagnosis of tubal pregnancy, making management more proactive.
+ Vaginal ultrasound, combined with the use of sensitive blood and urine tests that detect the presence of human chorionic gonadotrophin, helps to ensure earlier diagnosis.

- If the tube ruptures, shock may ensue; therefore resuscitation followed by laparotomy is needed.
- The mother should be offered follow-up support and information regarding subsequent pregnancies.

Further reading

National Institute for Health and Care Excellence, 2012. Ectopic pregnancy and miscarriage: diagnosis and initial management. Clinical guideline 154. https://www.nice.org.uk/guidance/cg154.
The Ectopic Pregnancy Trust. Clinical features of an ectopic pregnancy. http://www.ectopic.org.uk/professionals/clinical-features/.

Erythema toxicum

Erythema toxicum is a rash consisting of white papules on an erythematous base. It occurs in about 30%–70% of infants. The condition is benign and should not be confused with a staphylococcal infection, which will require antibiotics. Diagnosis can be confirmed by microscopic examination of a smear of aspirate from a pustule, which will show numerous eosinophils (white cells indicative of an allergic response rather than infection).

Further reading

Payne, J., 2016. Erythema toxicum neonatorum. Professional reference. http://patient.info/doctor/erythema-toxicum-neonatorum-pro.
Purvis, D., 2011. Toxic erythema of the newborn. DermNet NZ. https://www.dermnetnz.org/topics/toxic-erythema-of-the-newborn.

External cephalic version

External cephalic version (ECV) (Figs 10–12) is the use of external manipulation on the pregnant woman's abdomen to convert a breech (or transverse) to a cephalic presentation.

ECV may be offered at term but should only be undertaken in a unit where there are facilities for emergency delivery. Contraindications include:

- preeclampsia or hypertension
- multiple pregnancy

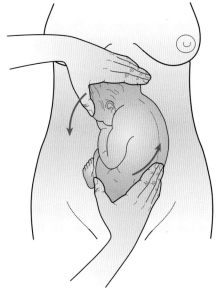

Fig. 10 The right hand lifts the breech out of the pelvis. The left hand makes the head follow the nose. Flexion of the head and back is maintained throughout.

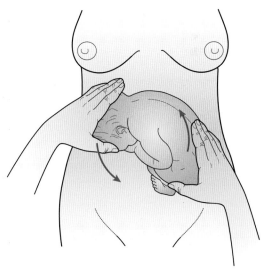

Fig. 11 Flexion is continued. The left hand brings the head downwards. The right hand pushes the breech upwards.

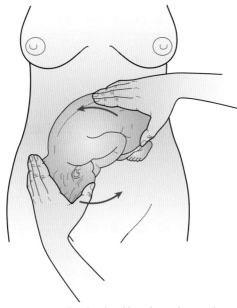

Fig. 12 Pressure is exerted on head and breech simultaneously until the head is lying at the pelvic brim.

- oligohydramnios (too little amniotic fluid)
- ruptured membranes
- a hydrocephalic fetus
- any condition that would require delivery by caesarean section

Further reading

Royal College of Obstetricians and Gynaecologists, 2017. External cephalic version and reducing the incidence of breech presentation. Green-top guideline no. 20a. https://www.rcog.org.uk/en/guidelines-research-services/guidelines/gtg20a/.

Female genital mutilation

The World Health Organization (WHO) defines female genital mutilation (FGM) as 'all procedures involving the partial or total removal of the external female genitalia or other injury to the female genital organs for non-medical reasons'.

The practice entails the removal and/or damaging of normal female genital tissue and can interfere with the normal function of the female body.

There are four types of FGM (Fig. 13), all of which are illegal in the UK.

Type 1. Clitoridectomy: Partial or total excision of the clitoris, and in a few cases of the prepuce only.

Type 2. Excision: Partial or complete excision of the clitoris and labia minora, with or without the removal of the labia majora.

Type 3. Infibulation: Narrowing of the vaginal opening by forming a covering seal by cutting and repositioning the inner or outer labia. It may also involve removal of the clitoris. This is the most extreme physical type and tends to lead to the most physical complications for the woman or girl, and at childbirth.

Type 4. Other: This type of FGM entails all other harmful practices to the female external genitalia for non-medical reasons, including pricking, piercing, incising, scraping and cauterizing. Type 4 includes labial stretching, as well as genital tattooing and piercing.

FGM is not associated with any health advantages and may lead to physical and psychological complications, and, in the worst cases, death of a woman or girl who has had FGM and/or death of her child due to complications in pregnancy and/or labour. FGM may be performed at any age, though the peak prevalence is five to eight years of age. In addition, women may undergo the procedure repeatedly after each time they give birth to restore the narrow vaginal opening created by type 3 FGM and widened in childbirth. This is called reinfibulation.

The practice of FGM is deeply rooted in certain cultures and communities. It is often viewed as a rite of passage performed to ensure that girls and young women remain pure and chaste in preparation for marriage. Other motives include hygiene, aesthetics, and religious and cultural reasons.

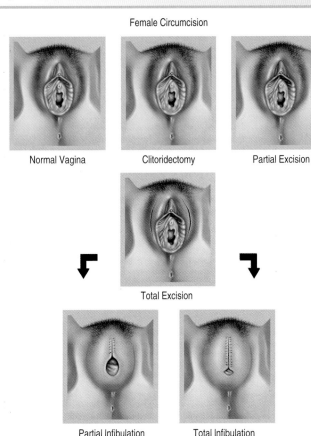

Fig. 13 **Types of female genital mutilation.**

It is, however, important to highlight that there is no basis for the practice of FGM in Muslim, Christian or Jewish religious texts.

FGM has been illegal in the UK since the Female Circumcision Act of 1985. The 1985 Act was superseded by the Female Genital Mutilation Act of 2003, which extended the offence to FGM performed abroad, and which makes FGM punishable by up to 14 years in prison. The Serious Crime Act 2015 introduced new provisions to tackle FGM, including the Mandatory Reporting Duty. Failure to comply may result in *Fitness to Practise* proceedings.

Further reading

Department of Health, 2015. Female genital mutilation (FGM): guidance for healthcare staff. (Collection of resources and guidance, updated 2017). https://www.gov.uk/government/collections/female-genital-mutilation-fgm-guidance-for-healthcare-staff.

HM Government, 2016. Multi-agency statutory guidance on female genital mutilation: https://www.gov.uk/government/uploads/system/uploads/attachment_data/file/512906/Multi_Agency_Statutory_Guidance_on_FGM__-_FINAL.pdf.

The Home Office, e-learning module on FGM. https://www.fgmelearning.co.uk (Need to register to access page.).

Royal College of Obstetricians and Gynaecologists, 2015. Female genital mutilation management. Green-top guideline no. 53. https://www.rcog.org.uk/en/guidelines-research-services/guidelines/gtg53/.

Royal College of Midwives, 2013. Tackling FGM in the UK: intercollegiate recommendations for identifying, recording and reporting. https://www.rcog.org.uk/globalassets/documents/news/tackingfgmuk.pdf.

WHO, 2016. Female genital mutilation. http://www.who.int/mediacentre/factsheets/fs241/en/.

Ferguson reflex

Surge of oxytocin, resulting in increased contractions, as the presenting part of the fetus stimulates nerve receptors in the pelvic floor, the cervix and upper portion of the vagina. As a consequence, the woman experiences the urge to push. This reflex becomes increasingly compulsive, overwhelming and involuntary. The woman's response is to employ secondary powers of expulsion by contracting her abdominal muscles and diaphragm.

Fetal alcohol syndrome

Congenital malformations associated with the mother's heavy consumption of alcohol during pregnancy. These include restricted growth, facial abnormalities, and learning and behavioural disorders, which are long lasting and may be lifelong. Other conditions that may arise from exposure to alcohol include cerebral palsy, epilepsy, learning disorders, behavioural problems, problems with liver, kidneys, heart or other organisms, hearing and sight problems, and a weakened immune system.

Some children may develop only mild signs or symptoms, whereas other may be severely affected.

Fetal alcohol spectrum disorder (FASD) is used to describe the condition associated with alcohol intake in pregnancy where the characteristics of fetal alcohol syndrome (FAS) are not fully manifested. No 'dose' of alcohol is known to be safe in pregnancy, so current advice is that women should abstain completely from drinking alcohol while trying to conceive and during pregnancy. Women who find it difficult to limit or exclude alcohol should be offered referral to local counselling or support services.

Further reading

Department of Health, 2016. UK Chief Medical Officers' Low Risk Drinking Guidelines. https://www.gov.uk/government/uploads/system/uploads/attachment_data/file/545937/UK_CMOs__report.pdf.

FASD Trust. (Support for those affected by FASD, and training/information for healthcare professionals.) http://www.fasdtrust.co.uk.

Fetal blood sampling

The use of fetal blood sampling (FBS) as part of screening for fetal anomalies has declined in recent years because improved molecular and cytogenic techniques allow more diagnoses to be made from chorionic villi or amniotic fluid. However, fetal blood may be advantageous when there are ambiguous findings from placental tissue. When there is rhesus isoimmunization it may be necessary to determine the fetal haemoglobin, in case intrauterine transfusion is required. Blood can be sampled from the umbilical cord or intrahepatic umbilical vein. In uncomplicated procedures after 20 weeks, FBS is associated with a 1% risk of miscarriage.

FBS is also used in conjunction with electronic fetal monitoring. When the fetal heart rate pattern is suspicious or pathological and fetal acidosis is suspected, FBS should always be carried out. A blood sample is taken from the fetal scalp via an amnioscope passed through the cervix (Fig. 14), and measurement of lactate or pH should be performed. An FBS pH result of ≤7.25 (lactate ≤4.1) is 'normal' but should be repeated within 30 minutes to 1 hour. An FBS pH <7.20 (lactate ≤4.9) indicates that the baby should be delivered.

Further reading

National Institute for Health and Care Excellence Pathways. Fetal blood sampling during labour (part of intrapartum care). http://pathways.nice.org.uk/pathways/intrapartum-care/fetal-blood-sampling-during-labour.

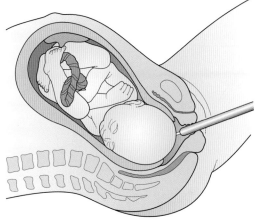

Fig. 14 Access to fetal scalp via amnioscope passed through the cervix.

Fontanelles

Fontanelles are membrane-covered 'soft spots' in the spaces where two sutures in the fetal skill join together. They allow for growth of the brain and skull during the baby's first year of life.

The posterior fontanelle usually closes by the time the baby is 1–3 months old. The anterior fontanelle usually closes between 7 and 19 months.

Fontanelles should feel firm and very slightly curved inward to the touch. A tense or bulging fontanelle may indicate increased intracranial pressure. Possible causes include encephalitis, hydrocephalus or meningitis.

A sunken fontanelle may indicate dehydration or malnutrition.

Midwives should check the size and tension of the fontanelles as part of a discharge examination, which should include occipitofrontal circumference (OFC), suture lines, cranial moulding, caput succedaneum and cephalohaematoma. Any abnormalities should be reported to a senior paediatrician and documented in the baby's case notes.

Forceps delivery

Forceps delivery (Figs 15–18) is one of the alternatives (the other being ventouse) for assisted or operative (instrumental) vaginal delivery, used when the mother is unable to give birth without medical or surgical assistance. Assisted vaginal birth is a widely practised intervention, accounting for approximately 11% of births in the UK, and 15% in Australia and

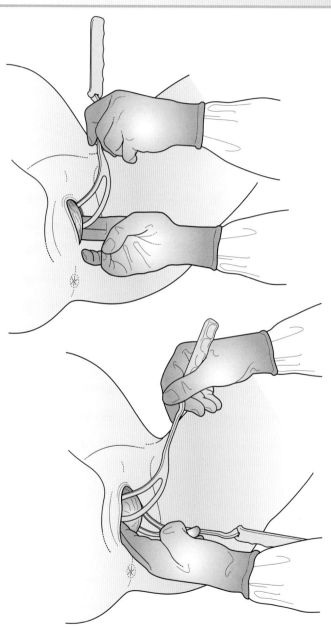

Figs 15–18 Technique for forceps delivery.

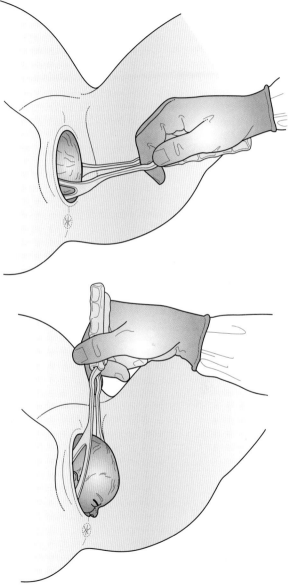

Figs 15–18, cont'd

Canada. Women who use epidural analgesia are at increased risk of having an instrumental assisted birth.

Forceps are most commonly used to expedite the birth of the head, or to protect the fetus or the mother, or both, from trauma and exhaustion. Forceps are also used to assist the delivery of the after-coming head of the breech.

Obstetric forceps are composed of two separate blades, right and left, that are inserted separately on each side of the head and then locked together. The blades are spoon shaped (cephalic curve) to accommodate the form of the baby's head.

Forceps deliveries fall into two categories, low and mid-cavity. High cavity forceps are now considered unsafe and a caesarean section will be carried out instead.

The main indications for a forceps delivery are delay in the second stage of labour, fetal compromise and maternal distress.

Prior to forceps delivery ensure:

+ the woman's bladder is empty to prevent injury
+ adequate analgesia is provided (epidural or pudendal block plus perineal infiltration of local anaesthetic)
+ information is given and consent obtained
+ paediatrician or advanced neonatal practitioner is informed and available if required
+ neonatal resuscitation equipment is checked and prepared in case it is necessary

Further reading

Royal College of Obstetricians and Gynaecologists, 2011. Operative vaginal delivery. Green-top guideline no. 26. https://www.rcog.org.uk/globalassets/documents/guidelines/gtg_26.pdf.

Fundal height

The fundal height (Fig. 19) is the distance between the top part of the uterus (the fundus) and the symphysis pubis (the junction between the pubic bones). Measurement of fundal height is undertaken to assess the increasing size of the uterus antenatally and decreasing size postnatally.

Assessing uterine size to compare it with gestation does not always produce an accurate result. If the uterus is unduly big the fetus may be

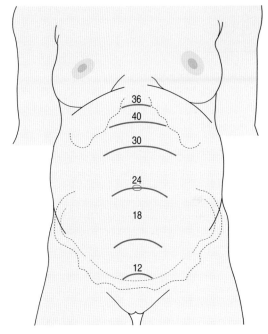

Fig. 19 Fundal height.

large or it may indicate multiple pregnancies or polyhydramnios. When the uterus is smaller than expected the last menstrual period (LMP) may be incorrect, or the fetus may be small for gestational age. Further investigation is warranted.

Resources

Perinatal Institute. Fetal growth—fundal height measurements. https://www.perinatal.org.uk/fetalgrowth/FundalHeight.aspx.
Perinatal Institute. Fetal growth examples. https://www.perinatal.org.uk/FetalGrowth/Examples.aspx.

German measles See Rubella.

Gestational diabetes

Gestational diabetes is any degree of glucose intolerance with its onset or first diagnosis during pregnancy, and usually resolving shortly after delivery. It is thought that hormones associated with pregnancy increase postprandial glucose concentrations and insulin resistance. This is normally countered by an increase in insulin production, but in gestational diabetes the compensatory rise is insufficient. Gestational diabetes usually develops in the third trimester.

Up to 5% of women giving birth in the UK have either preexisting diabetes or gestational diabetes. Of women who have diabetes during pregnancy, it is estimated that approximately 87.5% have gestational diabetes (which may or may not resolve after pregnancy), 7.5% have type 1 diabetes and the remaining 5% have type 2 diabetes. The prevalence of type 1 diabetes and especially type 2 diabetes, has increased in recent years. The incidence of gestational diabetes is also increasing as a result of higher rates of obesity in the general population and more pregnancies in older women.

Diabetes in pregnancy is associated with risks to the woman and to the developing fetus. Miscarriage, preeclampsia and preterm labour are more common in women with preexisting diabetes. In addition, diabetic retinopathy can worsen rapidly during pregnancy. Stillbirth, congenital malformations, macrosomia, birth injury, perinatal mortality and postnatal adaptation problems (such as hypoglycaemia) are more common in babies born to women with preexisting diabetes.

The risk of developing gestational diabetes is assessed using risk factors in a healthy population. At the initial assessment, determine the following:

- BMI (body mass index) above 30 kg/m^2
- previous macrosomic baby weighing 4.5 kg or more
- previous gestational diabetes
- family history of diabetes (first degree relative)
- minority ethnic family origin with a high prevalence of diabetes

The National Institute for Health and Care Excellence (NICE) guideline states fasting plasma glucose, random blood glucose, HbA1c, glucose challenge test or urinalysis for glucose should *not* be used to assess risk of developing gestational diabetes.

Gestational diabetes is diagnosed if the woman has a fasting plasma glucose level of 5.6 mmol/L or above, or a 2-hour plasma glucose level of 7.8 mmol/L or above.

Management is initially with dietary and lifestyle changes but if these have not reduced blood glucose to acceptable levels (less than 7.0 mmol/L) within 1–2 weeks, treatment should be with metformin and/or insulin. Treatment should be discontinued immediately after delivery, but women should have a fasting plasma glucose test 6–13 weeks after birth to exclude diabetes.

Women with gestational diabetes should give birth no later than 40+6 weeks, and should be offered induction of labour or caesarean section if they have not delivered by this time.

Further reading

NICE, 2015. Diabetes in pregnancy: management from preconception to the postnatal period. NG3. https://www.nice.org.uk/guidance/ng3.

Tidy, C., 2016. Gestational diabetes (professional reference). http://patient.info/doctor/gestational-diabetes.

Group B streptococcus

Group B streptococcus (GBS) is the leading cause of serious neonatal infection in the UK, and affects between 0.5/1000 and 1.15/1000 live births.

GBS is a gram-positive bacterium that naturally colonizes the genital and gastrointestinal tracts, and is carried asymptomatically by up to 40% of adults. It is not considered to be a sexually transmitted disease but infection increases with sexual activity and rates are highest among women attending genitourinary medicine clinics.

In pregnant women colonized with GBS, there is a high risk of pre-term delivery, prolonged rupture of membranes or maternal pyrexia during labour, and risk of vertical transmission to the baby. GBS is able to infiltrate the amniotic cavity, whether or not the membranes are intact, and infect the fetus. Postpartum endometritis and postcaesarean wound infection may also occur in the mother.

In the USA, pregnant women are screened in the third trimester and treated prophylactically if identified as high risk of transmitting the infection. However, routine screening in the UK is not considered clinically effective or cost-effective.

Further reading

Royal College of Obstetricians and Gynaecologists, 2012. The prevention of early-onset neonatal group B streptococcal disease. Green-top guideline no. 36. https://www.rcog.org.uk/globalassets/documents/guidelines/gtg_36.pdf.

H

Haemolytic disease of the newborn

Haemolytic disease of the newborn (HDN) is the immune-mediated red cell breakdown that occurs in rhesus disease and ABO incompatibility (not to be confused with haemorrhagic disease of the newborn—vitamin K deficiency bleeding). The majority of HDN is caused by the rhesus D antigen, which can cross the placenta and attach to fetal red blood cells. These cells are then destroyed by the fetus' immune system (haemolysis), resulting in anaemia, hyperbilirubinemia and excessive erythroid tissue in the liver, spleen, bone marrow, skin and placenta. In severe cases, multi-organ failure may occur.

HDN is much less common since the introduction of anti-D prophylaxis.

Antenatally, the first indication of HDN is the presence of anti-D antibodies in the mother's blood (see Coombs test). Routine ultrasound may detect hydrops fetalis or polyhydramnios.

Fetal blood sampling should be considered if a Doppler scan of the middle cerebral artery suggests anaemia. If confirmed, management is by transfusion via the umbilical vein.

Infants born to alloimmunized mothers may appear clinically normal in mild cases, but should be monitored closely for signs of late anaemia due to ongoing haemolysis. Signs and symptoms include lethargy, pallor and poor feeding history. It is not unusual for a baby to develop a severe anaemia requiring blood transfusion.

Further reading

Waggle, S., 2016. Hemolytic disease of newborn. Medscape. http://emedicine.medscape.com/article/974349-overview.

Haemorrhage

Haemorrhage is literally the escape of blood from any blood vessel. In pregnancy, the two main types of haemorrhage of particular concern are antepartum haemorrhage (APH) and postpartum haemorrhage (PPH).

Antepartum haemorrhage

Antepartum haemorrhage is bleeding from the genital tract after the 24th week of gestation and before the onset of labour (Table 4). If the bleeding is severe it may be accompanied by shock and disseminated intravascular coagulation (DIC). It can be fatal or result in permanent ill health. Fetal mortality and morbidity are also increased as a result of severe vaginal bleeding in pregnancy. Stillbirth or neonatal death may occur. Premature placental separation and consequent hypoxia may result in severe neurological damage to the baby.

APH is unpredictable and the woman's condition can deteriorate rapidly. A rapid decision about the urgency of need for a medical or paramedic presence or both must be made while observing the woman:

- take a history
- observe pulse rate, respiratory rate, blood pressure and temperature

Table 4 **Causes and incidence of bleeding in late pregnancy**

Cause	Incidence (%)
Placenta praevia	31
Placental abruption	22
'Unclassified', e.g.,	47
Marginal	
Show	
Cervicitis	
Trauma	
Vulvovaginal varicosities	
Genital tumours	
Genital infections	
Haematuria	
Vasa praevia	
Other	

- assess amount of blood lost
- perform a gentle abdominal examination, observing for signs that the woman is going into labour
- *on no account must any vaginal or rectal examination be done; nor may an enema or suppository be given to a woman suffering from APH*

Fetal condition

- Ask the mother if the baby has been moving as much as usual.
- Attempt to auscultate the fetal heart; ultrasound apparatus may be used.

Diagnosis

Pain—did the pain precede bleeding and is it continuous or intermittent?

Onset of bleeding—was it associated with any event such as abdominal trauma or sexual intercourse?

Amount of visible blood loss—is there any reason to suspect some blood has been retained in utero?

Colour of the blood—bright red or dark?

Consistency of the abdomen—soft or tense and board-like?

Tenderness of the abdomen—does the woman tense on examination palpation?

Lie, presentation and engagement—are any of these abnormal taking account of parity and gestation?

Audibility of fetal heart—is the fetal heart heard?

Ultrasound scan—does a scan suggest that the placenta is in the lower uterine segment?

See also Placenta praevia.

Further reading

National Institute for Health and Care Excellence, 2014. Intrapartum care for healthy women and babies. Clinical guideline (CG190). https://www.nice.org.uk/guidance/cg190.

Royal College of Obstetricians & Gynaecologists, 2011. Antepartum haemorrhage (Green-top guideline No 63). https://www.rcog.org.uk/globalassets/documents/guidelines/gtg_63.pdf.

Postpartum haemorrhage

PPH is defined as excessive bleeding from the genital tract at any time following the baby's birth, up to 12 weeks after birth.

Primary PPH occurs during the third stage of labour or within 24 hours of delivery. A measured loss that reaches 500 mL or any loss that adversely affects the mother constitutes a PPH. There are several reasons why PPH may occur, including:

+ atonic uterus
+ retained placenta
+ trauma
+ blood coagulation disorder

Signs may be obvious, such as visible bleeding or maternal collapse, but more subtle signs may present, including:

+ pallor
+ rising pulse rate
+ falling blood pressure
+ altered level of consciousness
+ an enlarged uterus that feels 'boggy' on palpation, i.e., soft, distended and lacking tone, even if little visible blood loss

Prophylaxis

+ Identify risk factors antenatally (high parity, presence of fibroids, maternal anaemia, ketoacidosis, multiple pregnancy)
+ Prevent prolonged labour and ketoacidosis
+ Ensure the mother does not have a full bladder at any stage
+ Administer a uterotonic agent
+ If a woman is known to have a placenta praevia, keep two units of cross matched blood available

Management of postpartum haemorrhage

The three principles of care:

+ call for medical aid
+ stop the bleeding
    + rub up a contraction
    + give a uterotonic
    + empty the bladder
    + empty the uterus
    + apply pressure if there is trauma
+ resuscitate the mother

Secondary postpartum haemorrhage

Secondary PPH is excessive or prolonged vaginal loss from 24 hours after delivery and for up to 12 weeks postpartum. Regardless of the timing of any haemorrhage it is most frequently the placental site that is the source. Alternatively, a cervical or deep vaginal wall tear, or trauma to the perineum might be the cause in women who have recently given birth. Retained placental fragments or other products of conception are likely to inhibit the process of involution, or reopen the placental wound. Diagnosis is likely to be determined by the woman's condition and the pattern of events, and is often complicated by the presence of infection.

Signs of secondary postpartum haemorrhage

- Lochial loss is heavier than usual
- Lochia returns to a bright red loss and may be offensive
- Subinvolution of the uterus
- Pyrexia and tachycardia
- Haematoma formation

Treatment

- Call a doctor
- Rub up a contraction by massaging the uterus if it is still palpable
- Express any clots
- Encourage the woman to empty her bladder
- Give a uterotonic drug intravenously or by intramuscular injection
- Keep all pads and linen to assess volume of blood lost
- Antibiotics may be prescribed
- If retained products of conception are seen on an ultrasound scan, surgery may be required

---

Further reading

Harding, M., 2015. Postpartum haemorrhage. (Professional reference.) http://patient.info/doctor/postpartum-haemorrhage.

Royal College of Obstetricians and Gynaecologists, 2009, revised April 2011. Postpartum haemorrhage, prevention and management. Green-top guideline No 52. https://www.rcog.org.uk/en/guidelines-research-services/guidelines/gtg52/.

Healthcare associated infections

Healthcare associated infections (HCAIs) can develop either as a direct result of healthcare interventions such as medical or surgical treatment, or from being in contact with a healthcare setting.

HCAI covers a wide range of infections, including those caused by methicillin-resistant *Staphylococcus aureus* (MRSA) and *Clostridium difficile* (C. difficile). Other more common types of HCAI are respiratory tract infections, urinary tract infections, surgical site infections, sepsis, gastro-intestinal infections and bloodstream infections.

HCAIs pose a serious risk to patients, staff and visitors; they cause significant morbidity to those infected and incur significant costs to healthcare providers.

The prevalence of HCAIs in hospitals in England alone in 2011 was 6.4% (National Institute for Health and Care Excellence [NICE], 2011).

Prevention and control are fundamental to improve the quality and safety of care provided to patients.

In maternity services, women most at risk are those who have a caesarean section or other invasive procedure. It is therefore essential to practise aseptic non-touch techniques (ANTT) whenever a procedure bypasses the body's natural defences (i.e., the skin or mucous membranes), for example, procedures such as cannulation, venipuncture, administration of intravenous drugs, wound care, urinary catheterization etc. Hand hygiene is the leading measure for reducing HCAIs.

Further reading

NICE, 2011. Healthcare-associated infections: prevention and control. Public health guideline PH36. https://www.nice.org.uk/guidance/ph36.

Haemorrhagic disease of the newborn See Vitamin K deficiency bleeding (VKDB).

Heart disease

Heart disease is the leading nonobstetric cause of maternal death in the UK. The most common cardiac cause of maternal death is myocardial infarction. The total incidence of cardiac disease in pregnancy is 0.5%–2%. Signs and symptoms of cardiac disease include:

+ dyspnoea
+ chest pain
+ limitation of activity
+ palpitations, arrhythmias, dysrhythmias
+ cyanosis
+ heart sound changes

During pregnancy, women with preexisting heart disease may experience a worsening of symptoms due to physiological changes of pregnancy—increase in circulating blood volume, increased resting oxygen consumption, decreased peripheral vascular resistance, increase in stroke volume and slight increase in resting heart rate. These changes influence haemodynamics, increasing strain on the heart, which is further compromised during labour. Maternal heart disease may be congenital or acquired.

The fetus is at increased risk of:

+ congenital cardiac defects
+ intrauterine hypoxia
+ intrauterine death
+ effects of maternal medication

Antenatal care

Prepregnancy counselling and then care in a dedicated antenatal cardiac clinic are required, with input from an obstetrician, cardiologist, anaesthetist and midwife. The aims of antenatal care are to detect heart failure and disturbances of cardiac rhythm. A high protein, low carbohydrate, low salt diet is recommended; weight control is important. Infections (including dental infections) should be treated with antibiotics to reduce the risk of bacterial endocarditis. Major antenatal complications are acute pulmonary oedema and congestive cardiac failure. Symptoms of a worsening of the condition (dyspnoea, cough or chest pain) indicate the need for immediate hospital admission.

Care in labour

Depending on the condition and progress of the pregnancy, labour may be spontaneous or induced, or an elective caesarean section may be carried out. Prophylactic antibiotics may be given to reduce the risk of bacterial endocarditis. Epidural analgesia is recommended but with caution in respect of hypotension, and is contraindicated in women on anticoagulant therapy.

In addition to usual midwifery observations, the following are important:

+ colour in case of cyanosis
+ respiratory rate—should remain below 24 per minute
+ degree of dyspnoea
+ radial and apical pulses—should remain below 110 per minute
+ electrocardiogram (ECG) may be continuous throughout labour
+ fluid balance to prevent overload
+ continuous electronic fetal monitoring

There is no reason for instrumental delivery if birth is progressing well, but excessive pushing should be avoided. Strong uterine contraction in the third stage may alter circulation and compromise an impaired heart: ergometrine and ergometrine/oxytocin are not used, and oxytocin used with caution (contraindicated in heart failure).

Postnatal care

Continue close observation of vital signs as heart failure or peripartum cardiomyopathy may occur in the first few days postnatally. Women require rest but not immobilization. Physiotherapy may reduce the risk of thromboembolic disorders. There is usually no contraindication to breastfeeding. Careful examination of the baby to exclude congenital heart disease (increased risk) is required.

Further reading

European Society of Cardiology, 2011. ESC Guidelines on the management of cardiovascular diseases during pregnancy. Eur. Heart J. 32, 3147–3197. Doi:10.1093/eurheartj/ehr218. https://www. escardio.org/static_file/Escardio/Guidelines/publications/ PREGN%20Guidelines-Pregnancy-FT.pdf.

Royal College of Obstetricians and Gynaecologists, 2011. Cardiac disease and pregnancy. Good practice no. 13. https://www.rcog. org.uk/globalassets/documents/guidelines/ goodpractice13cardiacdiseaseandpregnancy.pdf.

Haemolysis, elevated liver enzymes and low platelet count syndrome

The syndrome of haemolysis, elevated liver enzymes and low platelet count (HELLP) is considered a variant of preeclampsia/eclampsia. Pregnancies affected by this syndrome are associated with significant maternal and perinatal morbidity and mortality. HELLP syndrome typically presents between 32 and 34 weeks' gestation but 30% of cases occur postpartum.

Signs

+ Sharp rise in blood pressure
+ Diminished urinary output
+ Increase in proteinuria
+ Headache: usually severe, persistent and frontal in location
+ Drowsiness or confusion
+ Visual disturbances, e.g., blurring of vision or flashing lights
+ Epigastric pain
+ Nausea and vomiting

Women with HELLP syndrome should be admitted to a consultant unit with intensive or high dependency facilities. In pregnancies of less than 32 weeks' gestation, expectant management may be undertaken with appropriate safeguards and consent. In term pregnancies, or where there is a deteriorating maternal or fetal condition, immediate delivery is recommended.

Further reading

Khan, H,. 2015. HELLP syndrome. Medscape. http://emedicine. medscape.com/article/1394126-overview.

Payne, J., 2016. HELLP syndrome. (Professional reference). http:// patient.info/doctor/hellp-syndrome.

Preeclampsia Foundation, 2015. HELLP syndrome. http://www. preeclampsia.org/health-information/hellp-syndrome.

Hepatitis

The hepatitis viruses A, B, C, D and E cause acute hepatitis. Hepatitis B and, particularly, C, can cause chronic infection that can lead to cirrhosis, liver failure and liver cancer. All types of viral hepatitis are notifiable diseases in UK.

Services will have a policy for vaccinations against hepatitis A and B. Acute infection may present with:

+ nausea and vomiting
+ myalgia
+ fatigue/malaise
+ right upper quadrant pain
+ change in sense of smell or taste
+ coryza
+ photophobia
+ headache

Diarrhoea (with pale stools) and dark urine may also be present. However, often there are no signs unless jaundice develops, when hepatomegaly, splenomegaly and lymphadenopathy may also occur.

Hepatitis A

Previously a common childhood infection in the UK but now unusual. May occur in outbreaks in institutions, and is common in travellers. Infection confers immunity. Spread normally by the faecal-oral route (ingestion of food or drink contaminated by infected stool) but occasionally through blood. Usually self-limiting (rarely fulminant); there is no carrier state, and chronic liver disease does not occur. HepA vaccine can protect people at high risk, e.g., those who have been in contact with an infected person, travellers to countries where the infection is common and injecting drug users.

Hepatitis B

Early symptoms are flu-like; infection can lead to liver disease and liver cancer. Hepatitis B is 10–100 times more infectious than HIV (Centers for disease control [CDC], 2016). Transmitted by contact with infected blood or body fluids, for example, by

- sharing or use of contaminated equipment during injecting drug use
- vertical transmission (mother to baby) from an infectious mother to her unborn child
- sexual transmission
- receipt of infectious blood (via transfusion) or infectious blood products (e.g., clotting factors)
- needlestick or other sharps injuries (in particular those sustained by healthcare workers)
- tattooing and body piercing

HepB vaccination

- Should be given to all individuals at risk, including health professionals
- Is usually provided free (on the NHS) to people in a high-risk group
- Is not free if requested for travel abroad

Hepatitis C

Often asymptomatic initially; 15%–20% clear their infection within 2–6 months (National Institute for Health and Care Excellence [NICE], 2016). Of those with chronic infection, some remain well but many develop mild to moderate liver damage (with or without symptoms); of these, 20% progress to cirrhosis over 20–30 years. Excessive alcohol consumption increases risk of severe liver complications. Hepatitis C is blood borne and most often acquired through injecting drug use; also by sharing razors or toothbrushes or during body piercing (e.g., tattooing, acupuncture) with nonsterile needles. It was also spread by blood transfusions before September 1991, when screening for hepatitis C was brought in. There is no vaccine. Increasingly effective drug treatment (not suitable for everyone, lasts 6 or 12 months) can clear the virus approximately 90% of the time. Around 214,000 people in the UK are thought to have chronic hepatitis C (NICE 2016); the Department of Health (DH) runs awareness campaigns to promote diagnosis and treatment.

Hepatitis D

An important cause of acute and severe chronic liver damage in some parts of the world (Mediterranean, parts of Eastern Europe, Middle East, Africa and South America). Occurs only in people already infected with hepatitis B.

Hepatitis E

Uncommon in the UK, but common in Asia, Africa and Central America, particularly where sanitation is poor. Disease is usually mild but, rarely, can be fatal, particularly in pregnant women. Transmission and clinical features are similar to those of hepatitis A.

Further reading

CDC, 2016. Viral hepatitis—hepatitis B information. http://www.cdc.gov/hepatitis/hbv/bfaq.htm.

Henderson, R., 2016. Hepatitis B. Professional reference. http://www.patient.co.uk/doctor/hepatitis-b-pro.

Newson, L., 2016. Hepatitis A. Professional reference. http://www.patient.co.uk/doctor/hepatitis-a-pro.

NICE, 2016. Clinical Knowledge Summaries. Hepatitis C. http://cks.nice.org.uk/hepatitis-c.

Tidy, C., 2014. Chronic hepatitis. Professional reference. http://www.patient.co.uk/doctor/chronic-hepatitis.

Herpes

Herpes simplex virus (HSV) infection

Herpes labialis (cold sores)—localized collection of blisters with a red base, usually on or around the lips, that develop into crusts and disappear without scarring. Manifestation of a recurring infection with the herpes simplex virus (HSV), usually but not exclusively HSV-1. Lesions are contagious until dried out.

Genital herpes is almost exclusively a sexually transmitted infection, generally caused by HSV-2, although the prevalence of genital HSV-1 is increasing. Most transmission occurs via sexual contact with an individual who may be asymptomatic but is still shedding the virus. There is some evidence that genital HSV increases the risk of acquiring (and transmitting) HIV infection.

Genital herpes in pregnancy

See Sexually transmitted infections.

Further reading

Harding, M., 2015. Genital herpes in pregnancy. Professional reference. http://www.patient.co.uk/doctor/genital-herpes-in-pregnancy.

Harding, M., 2015. Herpes simplex genital. Professional reference. http://www.patient.co.uk/doctor/herpes-simplex-genital.

Herpes zoster virus infection

Chickenpox

Highly contagious infection with the varicella-zoster herpesvirus, usually affecting children. An attack gives lifelong immunity, but the virus remains dormant in nerves and in later life may cause shingles (see Shingles) Causes crops of itchy vesicles, typically starting on the back. Spread by direct contact or the respiratory route, via droplets. Seek advice if chickenpox exposure or infection occurs during pregnancy or if neonatal infection.

Shingles

Rash caused by reactivation of the dormant chickenpox (varicella zoster) virus, often many years after original infection. The condition can be painful and last a long time, and in some patients postherpetic neuralgia can develop or persist more than 90 days after the onset of the rash. Shingles is not infectious, but a person who has never had chickenpox may become infected with chickenpox from a person with shingles. Unlike chickenpox, shingles in pregnancy does not cause harm to the unborn baby, but should always be referred to a specialist as the benefits of antiviral treatments must be balanced against the possible risk of damage to the fetus.

HIV

HIV is a retrovirus that infects T helper lymphocytes, cells that coordinate the actions of other immune system cells and carry the CD4 receptor. Without treatment, over time the patient's CD4 count declines, susceptibility to infections increases, symptoms develop and become more severe until a diagnosis of acquired immune deficiency syndrome (AIDS) is made.

HIV is associated with significant mortality, serious morbidity and high costs of treatment and care. Around 100,000 people are living with HIV infection (diagnosed and undiagnosed) in the UK. The infection is still frequently regarded as stigmatizing, and has a prolonged 'silent' period during which it often remains undiagnosed.

Anti-retroviral therapy (ART) has resulted in substantial reductions in both the number of people who progress to AIDS and the number of AIDS-related deaths in the UK. People diagnosed promptly with HIV and started on ART early can expect near normal life expectancy. The number of circulating viruses (viral load) predicts progression to late-stage HIV disease.

HIV in pregnancy

All pregnant women are recommended screening for HIV infection, as well as syphilis, hepatitis B and rubella (see Rubella) in every pregnancy at their booking antenatal visit. In 2013, 2.5 pregnant women per 1000 were HIV-positive and the majority had been diagnosed before pregnancy. Without intervention, between 15% and 45% of babies born to HIV-infected mothers in the most severely affected parts of the world are also infected, but with appropriate interventions, mother-to-child (vertical) transmission rates can be reduced to less than 1%.

Interventions include ART, elective caesarean section (unless viral load is very low [less than 50 copies/mL]) and avoidance of breastfeeding after delivery.

Further reading

Knott, L., 2016. Human immunodeficiency virus (Professional reference). http://www.patient.co.uk/doctor/human-immunodeficiency-virus-hiv.

Knott, L., 2015. Management of HIV in pregnancy (Professional reference). http://patient.info/doctor/management-of-hiv-in-pregnancy.

Public Health England, 2014. HIV surveillance, data and management https://www.gov.uk/government/collections/hiv-surveillance-data-and-management.

Hyperemesis gravidarum

Excessive nausea and vomiting that starts between 4 and 10 weeks' gestation, resolves before 20 weeks and requires intervention is known as *hyperemesis gravidarum*. The woman presents with inability to retain food or fluids, leading to dehydration and malnourishment. She may have lost weight and be distressed and debilitated by her symptoms. Admission is required for assessment and management of symptoms:

- Hypovolaemia and electrolyte imbalance are corrected by intravenous infusion.
- Vitamin supplements can be given parenterally, particularly where hyperemesis has been prolonged.
- Initially nothing is given by mouth; fluids and diet are gradually reintroduced as the condition improves.
- Antiemetics may be prescribed.

Further reading

American Society of Obstetrics and Gynecology, 2015. Nausea and vomiting of pregnancy. Practice Bulletin Summary 153: Obstet. Gynecol. 126 (3), 687–688. http://journals.lww.com/greenjournal/Abstract/2015/09000/Practice_Bulletin_Summary_No_153_Nausea_and_Vomiting_of.42.aspx.

National Institute for Health and Care Excellence, 2013. Nausea/vomiting in pregnancy. Clinical Knowledge Summaries. http://cks.nice.org.uk/nauseavomiting-in-pregnancy.

Hyperglycaemia

Hyperglycaemia is less clinically significant that hypoglycaemia (see Hypoglycaemia) and occurs predominantly in preterm and severely growth-restricted infants. It is also seen in term infants in response to stress, especially following hypoxia-ischaemia, surgery or drugs such as corticosteroids. In general, no treatment is required.

Further reading

Sinclair, J.C., Bottino, M., Cowett, R.M., 2011. Interventions for prevention of neonatal hyperglycemia in very low birth weight infants. http://www.cochrane.org/CD007615/NEONATAL_interventions-for-prevention-of-neonatal-hyperglycemia-in-very-low-birth-weight-infants.

Hyperthermia

Hyperthermia is defined as a core temperature above 38°C. The usual cause is overheating of the environment but it can also be a clinical sign of sepsis, brain injury or drug therapy. Infants may attempt to regulate their temperature by increasing their respiratory rate, leading to increased fluid loss by evaporation through the airways. Hyperthermia may cause hypernatraemia, jaundice and recurrent apnoea.

Hypoglycaemia

A generally accepted definition of hypoglycaemia in infants is serum glucose of <2.6 mmol/L. Nonspecific signs in the newborn can be vague: they include lethargy, poor feeding and 'jitteriness'. These signs can also be due to sepsis and sometimes a healthy term infant can be sleepy and reluctant to feed. However, if these signs persist or worsen, the midwife should seek immediate paediatric advice and anticipate investigations for sepsis and hypoglycaemia. Specific signs comprise increasing lethargy and irritability with a reduction in level of consciousness and eventually seizures, associated with a risk of cerebral damage.

Be aware that reagent strips can be unreliable when blood glucose levels are very low, and a blood sample is required to provide a true blood (plasma) glucose level.

If low serum glucose is confirmed, urgent treatment is required to avoid permanent cerebral damage.

Risk factors for neurological sequelae of hypoglycaemia

+ Preterm infants (<37 weeks)
+ Growth restricted infants (<3rd centile for gestation)
+ Infants of diabetic mothers
+ Sick, term infants e.g., sepsis or following perinatal hypoxia-ischaemia
+ Infants with inborn errors of metabolism

Management

If serum glucose concentration is <2.6 mmol/L then feed should be given at increased volume and decreased frequency. Supplementary feeding with formula milk may be required in infants who are breastfed, and/or nasogastric tube (NGT) feeding—expressed breast milk can be used for NGT. In infants where enteral feeding is contraindicated for any reason intravenous 10% dextrose at 60 mL/kg per day should be initiated.

Further reading

Cranmer, H., 2014. Neonatal hypoglycemia. Medscape. http://emedicine.medscape.com/article/802334-overview.

Hypothermia

Hypothermia is defined as a core temperature below 36° C. This can cause complications such as:

+ increased oxygen consumption (due to thermogenesis from brown fat stores)
+ lactic acid production
+ apnoea
+ decrease in blood coagulability
+ hypoglycaemia (most common)

When neonates are exposed to cold they will at first become very restless, then, as their body temperature falls, they adopt a tightly flexed position to conserve heat. The sick or preterm infant will tend to lie supine in a frog-like position, which maximizes heat loss.

At birth a baby's temperature can fall very rapidly. The healthy term baby will try to maintain temperature within the normal range but for a baby compromised at birth the additional stress of hypothermia can be disastrous.

Unexplained hypothermia may be an indication of the onset of neonatal sepsis and must always trigger paediatric team involvement.

Hypoxia

Literally lack of oxygen, hypoxia in itself is initially the stimulus for the baby to take its first breath following birth. The majority of babies gasp and establish respiration within 60 seconds of birth. However, if they fail to do so, prompt resuscitation is needed. The length of time that the fetus or neonate is subjected to hypoxia determines the outcome.

Before birth

Oxygenation of the fetus is dependent on oxygenation of the mother, adequate perfusion of the placental site, fetoplacental circulation and adequate fetal haemoglobin. Absence or reduction of any of these factors will result in reduced oxygen supply to the fetus. The fetus responds to hypoxia by accelerating the heart rate in an effort to maintain supplies of oxygen to the brain. If hypoxia persists, cerebral blood vessels will dilate and some brain swelling may occur. As cardiac glycogen reserves are depleted, bradycardia develops, the anal sphincter relaxes and the fetus may pass meconium into the liquor. Gasping breathing movements triggered by hypoxia may result in aspiration of meconium-stained liquor into the lungs. Auscultation of the fetal heart, use of cardiotocography and observation of meconium staining of liquor draining from the vagina should alert the midwife to fetal compromise. Efforts should be made to expedite delivery.

After birth

In the neonate, the initial response to hypoxia is gasping respirations followed by a period of apnoea lasting $1\frac{1}{2}$ minutes—primary apnoea—which, if not resolved by intervention, is followed by a further episode of gasping respirations, which accelerate while diminishing in depth until, approximately 8 minutes after birth, respirations cease completely—secondary (terminal) apnoea. During primary apnoea, circulation and heart rate are maintained, and such babies respond quickly to simple resuscitation measures. In terminal apnoea, the circulation is impaired, heart rate is slow and the baby looks shocked.

The aims of resuscitation are to:

A.   Airway—open airway
B.   Breathing—inflate lungs and breathe for the baby
C.   Circulation—ensure effective circulation with chest compression if necessary
D.   Drugs—consider drugs to achieve this if initially unsuccessful

Do not allow the baby to get cold, and observe and record the sequence of events during resuscitation accurately.

Further reading

American Heart Association, 2010. Guidelines for cardiopulmonary resuscitation and emergency cardiovascular care science. Part 15: Neonatal resuscitation. Circulation, 122:S909-S919. http://circ.ahajournals.org/content/122/18_suppl_3/S909.full.

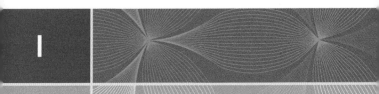

I

Induction of labour

Induction of labour is an intervention to stimulate uterine contractions before the onset of spontaneous labour.

Induction is indicated when the benefits to the mother or the fetus outweigh those of continuing the pregnancy. These include:

Maternal

+   Prolonged or postterm pregnancy
+   Hypertension, including preeclampsia
+   Diabetes
+   Medical problems, e.g., renal, respiratory or cardiac disease
+   Placental abruption
+   Obstetric history, such as previous stillbirth or previous caesarean section
+   Maternal request

Fetal

+ Suspected fetal compromise
+ Multiple pregnancy
+ Intrauterine death
+ Some breech presentations

Contraindications

+ Placenta praevia
+ Transverse or compound fetal presentation
+ Cephalopelvic disproportion
+ Severe fetal compromise
+ Active genital herpes

If delivery is imperative, it should be effected by caesarean section.

Methods of inducing labour

Prostaglandins

Before prescribing prostaglandin, assess cervix using the Bishop score (see Bishop score).

Prostaglandin preparations are available as gels, tablets or controlled-release pessaries. They are inserted close to the cervix, within the posterior fornix of the vagina. Fetal heart and uterine contractions should be monitored for 30–60 minutes thereafter.

Sweeping or stripping of membranes

Sweeping the membranes can be an effective method of inducing labour in an uncomplicated pregnancy. During a vaginal examination, the clinician inserts a finger through the cervical os, and using a sweeping or circular movement, releases the fetal membranes from the lower uterine segment. The woman should be made aware that this procedure may cause some discomfort and bleeding.

Amniotomy

Amniotomy is the artificial rupture of the fetal membranes (ARM) resulting in drainage of liquor. It is performed to induce labour when the cervix is favourable, or during labour to augment contractions. Amniotomy is also carried out to visualize the colour of the liquor or to attach a fetal scalp electrode for continuous electronic monitoring of the fetal heart rate.

Hazards include:

+ intrauterine infection
+ early deceleration of the fetal heart
+ cord prolapse

- bleeding from the fetal vessels in the membranes (vasa praevia), friable vessels in the cervix or placenta praevia

Oxytocin

Oxytocin is used in conjunction with ARM and may be commenced at the same time or after a delay of several hours. It is administered intravenously via a pump. The aim should be to use the lowest dose required to maintain effective, well-spaced contractions (maximum 3–4 contractions every 10 minutes). Oxytocin should not be started within 6 hours of administration of prostaglandins. Side effects include hyperstimulation of the uterus, which could cause fetal hypoxia and uterine rupture, and water retention; prolonged use may contribute to uterine atony postpartum.

Further reading

National Institute for Health and Care Excellence, 2008. Inducing labour. Clinical guideline 70. https://www.nice.org.uk/guidance/CG70.

World Health Organization, 2011. WHO recommendations for induction of labour: RHL review. The WHO Reproductive Health Library; Geneva: World Health Organization. http://www.who.int/reproductivehealth/publications/maternal_perinatal_health/9789241501156/en/.

Initial antenatal assessment

The purpose of the initial antenatal assessment (otherwise known as the booking[1] visit) is to:
- introduce the woman to the maternity service
- share information in order to discuss, plan and implement care for the duration of the pregnancy, the birth and postnatally

The earlier first contact is made with the midwife, the more appropriate and valuable the advice given relating to nutrition and care of the developing fetal organs. Medical conditions, infections, smoking, alcohol and drug taking may all have a profound and detrimental effect on the fetus at this time.

---

[1]The term 'booking' interview, although still used in practice, was originally used to describe the pregnant woman booking with her choice of maternity provider and booking in for her birth. This reflects the funding stream rather than the care required.

Among the topics to be covered are

+ social history
+ general health
+ menstrual history
+ obstetric history
+ medical history
+ family history

In addition to general observations, the midwife should undertake a physical examination, blood pressure, urinalysis and blood tests.

See Antenatal care; Antenatal Examination; Antenatal Screening.

Infertility

Infertility is defined as failure to conceive after regular unprotected intercourse for 12 months in the absence of known reproductive pathology. One in seven couples experience difficulty conceiving and may experience considerable psychological distress. The National Institute of Heath and Care Excellence (NICE) states that a woman of reproductive age who has not conceived after 1 year of unprotected vaginal sexual intercourse, in the absence of any known cause of infertility, should be offered further assessment and investigation (along with her partner), with earlier referral to a specialist if the woman is over 36 years of age.

Further reading

(NICE), 2013 (updated 2016). Fertility problems: assessment and treatment. Clinical guideline CG156. http://www.nice.org.uk/CG156.

Influenza/Influenza vaccination

Influenza is an acute viral infection of the respiratory tract. Of the three types of influenza virus (A, B and C), influenza A and B are responsible for most clinical illness. Influenza is characterized by the sudden onset of fever, chills, headache, myalgia and extreme fatigue. For otherwise healthy people, influenza is an unpleasant but generally self-limiting illness. However for certain groups—including pregnant women—there is a risk of more serious illness. Influenza during pregnancy may also be associated with perinatal mortality, prematurity, smaller neonatal size and lower birth weight.

Vaccination

All pregnant women are recommended to have the flu vaccine, irrespective of their stage of pregnancy. Inactivated vaccine can be administered safely during any trimester, and there has been no study to date that shows any increase in the risk of harm to the unborn baby or in maternal complications.

On the contrary, flu vaccination during pregnancy may reduce the likelihood of preterm birth and smaller infant size at birth, and it also offers some protection to the baby in its first few months of life.

Ideally, vaccine should be given before flu starts to circulate, but it is important that vaccination is offered to any woman who becomes pregnant during the flu season. The perfect time for this to take place is at the woman's first midwife appointment, but if the midwife is not an independent prescriber, the woman should be encouraged to attend her GP surgery for vaccination.

Further reading

Public Health England, 2015. Immunization against infectious disease. Influenza: the green book, chapter 19. https://www.gov.uk/government/publications/influenza-the-green-book-chapter-19.

Instrumental delivery See Operative vaginal delivery; Forceps; Ventouse method.

Intrauterine death

Intrauterine fetal death refers to babies with no signs of life in utero. Stillbirth is defined as a baby delivered with no signs of life, known to have died after 24 completed weeks of pregnancy. In the UK, 1 in 200 babies are stillborn each year. In 28% of stillbirths the cause remains unknown. Twelve per cent of stillbirths are attributed to placental conditions, 11% to antepartum/intrapartum haemorrhage and 9% to major congenital abnormality. Eight per cent of stillbirth deaths occur during labour or delivery.

Diagnosis

The mother may be aware of a decrease in fetal movements in many cases; others may be discovered at a routine antenatal check. Diagnosis is confirmed by ultrasound examination, which will reveal a lack of a visible heartbeat. Auscultation is insufficiently accurate for diagnosis, and may give false reassurance.

Delivery

Where the death is diagnosed antenatally, labour is induced using a combination of mifepristone and prostaglandin. While induction does not have to be immediate, it should take place within 2–3 days. Vaginal birth can be achieved within 24 hours of induction of labour in about 90% of women, but is often emotionally distressing, and the woman may opt for a caesarean birth. The implications of a caesarean section for future childbearing should be discussed.

The mother who has to deliver a stillborn baby requires significant psychological support. She may request substantial amount of pain relief, not realizing that later she may wish she could fully remember the birth of the baby.

Intrauterine death is a risk factor for the development of disseminated intravascular coagulation (DIC), which increases from low at 48 hours to 10% within 4 weeks. The woman's condition should be monitored carefully. After delivery blood should be taken for full blood count, clotting screen, Kleihauer test, HBA1c, cultures, serology and cytogenetics.

After the birth

After the baby is born, it is important to provide the mother and her partner with time—away from the normal postnatal ward—to spend with their baby and have the opportunity to hold it, to wash and dress the baby if they wish or to watch while a member of staff does so. It is also important to enable the parents to have mementoes of the baby, which may include photographs, the baby's name-band, foot and hand prints and a lock of hair.

Parents should be offered full postmortem examination to help explain the cause of an intrauterine fetal death, but should not be persuaded to accept the offer against their wishes, or cultural or religious beliefs. Consent must be obtained, even for less invasive tests.

Women should also be offered pharmacological measures to suppress lactation, to avoid physical discomfort and emotional distress.

All key staff groups must be informed to ensure cancellation of existing appointments and continuity of follow-up. Carers must be alert to the fact that women (and their partners and other children) are at risk of prolonged severe psychological reactions, including post-traumatic stress disorder.

Stillbirth must be medically certified by the doctor or midwife present at the birth or who examined the baby after birth, and the Coroner must be contacted if there is doubt about the status of the birth. Fetal deaths delivered later than 24 weeks that had clearly occurred before the end of the 24th week do not have to be certified or registered.

Caring for a woman with a stillbirth can take a heavy emotional toll on the midwife, and midwives also need effective support systems.

Further reading

Harding, M., 2014. Stillbirth and neonatal death. (Professional reference.) http://patient.info/doctor/stillbirth-and-neonatal-death.

Royal College of Obstetricians and Gynaecologists, 2010. Late intrauterine fetal death and stillbirth. Green-top guideline No 55. https://www.rcog.org.uk/globalassets/documents/guidelines/gtg_55.pdf.

SANDS, the Stillbirth and neonatal death charity. Further reading for professionals. http://www.uk-sands.org/professionals.

Intrauterine growth restriction

Failure of normal fetal growth caused by multiple adverse effects on the fetus.

Fetal growth is regulated by maternal, placental and fetal factors, any or all of which can be implicated in intrauterine growth restriction.

Asymmetric (acute) growth is when weight is reduced out of proportion to length and head circumference. It is thought to be caused by extrinsic factors such as pregnancy-induced hypertension.

+ Head looks disproportionately large in relation to body
+ Head circumference is usually within normal parameters
+ Bones are within gestational norms for length and density
+ Anterior fontanelle may be larger than expected
+ Abdomen looks sunken (due to shrinkage of liver and spleen)
+ Decreased fat deposition
+ Skin is loose and appears wizened or 'old'
+ Vernix caseosa is reduced or absent
+ Unless severely affected, these babies appear hyperactive and hungry

Symmetric (chronic) growth is due to decreased growth potential of the fetus as a result of congenital infection or chromosomal/genetic defects (intrinsic) or extrinsic factors occurring early in gestation (e.g., effects of maternal smoking or poor dietary intake).

+ Head circumference, length and weight are proportionately reduced for gestational age
+ Babies are diminutive in size
+ They do not appear wasted and have subcutaneous fat appropriate to their size
+ Skin is taut

- Babies are generally vigorous and less likely to be hypoglycaemic or polycythaemic
- They may suffer major congenital abnormalities and can be a source of infection to carers as a result of transplacental infection

Further reading

Goss, M., 2015. Fetal growth restriction. Medscape. http://emedicine.medscape.com/article/261226-overview.

Tidy, C., 2016. Intrauterine growth restriction. (Professional reference.) http://patient.info/doctor/intrauterine-growth-restriction.

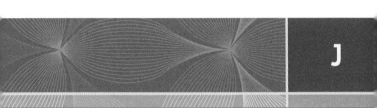

J

Jaundice

Jaundice occurs when bilirubin, a yellow pigment released when red blood cells are broken down, builds up in the blood. The skin and the whites of the eyes have a yellow tinge. Jaundice in adults and in older children usually indicates underlying disease. Neonatal jaundice is common. The indications for phototherapy vary between units. Refer for urgent hospital assessment if jaundice presents in the first 24 hours of life, the baby is jaundiced *and* unwell or for prolonged jaundice (more than 14 days in babies with gestational age of >37 weeks, or 21 days in those with gestational age of <37 weeks).

Jaundice in pregnancy

Jaundice in pregnancy, while relatively rare, has potentially serious consequences for maternal and fetal health.

Further reading

Henderson, R., 2015. Jaundice. Professional reference. https://patient.info/doctor/jaundice-pro.

Tidy, C., 2015. Jaundice in pregnancy. http://www.patient.co.uk/doctor/Jaundice-in-Pregnancy.htm.

Tidy, C., 2016. Neonatal jaundice. http://www.patient.co.uk/doctor/neonatal-jaundice-pro.

K

Karyotyping

Karyotyping is a test to examine chromosomes in a sample of cells. This test can help identify genetic causes of a disorder or disease. The test can be performed on almost any tissue, including amniotic fluid, blood, bone marrow or the placenta. Normal results will show, in females, 44 autosomes and 2 sex chromosomes (XX), and in males, 44 autosomes and 2 sex chromosomes (XY).

Kernicterus (bilirubin toxicity)

Kernicterus is a rare but serious complication of severe untreated jaundice in newborn babies, caused by excess bilirubin damaging the central nervous system by crossing the blood-brain barrier. It affects less than 1 in 100,000 babies in the UK.

Early signs include lethargy, decreased awareness of surroundings, loss of muscle tone (floppiness) and poor feeding. Late symptoms may include muscle rigidity, hyperextension of the neck or spine, or seizures.

Treatment is via exchange transfusion. If significant brain damage occurs before treatment the child may develop permanent disabilities including cerebral palsy, hearing loss and learning difficulties.

Further reading

Medline Plus, 2015. Bilirubin encephalopathy. https://www.nlm.nih.gov/medlineplus/ency/article/007309.htm.
NHS Choices, 2015. Kernicterus in newborn babies. http://www.nhs.uk/Conditions/Jaundice-newborn/Pages/Complications.aspx.

Ketoacidosis

Ketoacidosis is a life-threatening condition caused by a severe lack of insulin that can occur in type 1 and, less commonly, type 2, diabetes. Blood glucose is high, too little glucose enters cells and the body breaks down other body tissue (e.g., fat) as an energy source. Acidic ketones are produced, and will be detectable in the urine and blood. In pregnancy, ketoacidosis compromises both the fetus and the mother. The majority of cases occur in the second and third trimesters of pregnancy. It tends to occur at lower blood glucose levels and more rapidly than in non-pregnant women, often causing delay in diagnosis. Early detection of ketonuria is essential because ketoacidosis is a factor associated with intrauterine death, and its detection warrants immediate admission for intravenous fluids, insulin and medical review and monitoring.

Further reading

Kamalakannan, D., Baskar, V., Barton, D.M., Abdu, T.A.M., 2003. Diabetic ketoacidosis in pregnancy. Postgrad. Med. J. 79, 454–457. http://pmj.bmj.com/content/79/934/454.full.

Ketonuria

Ketones are formed as a result of metabolism of fatty acids when the body cannot access adequate calories from glucose (derived from carbohydrates) to meet energy requirements and fetal demands, for example, in hyperemesis gravidarum or gestational diabetes. In pregnancy, urinary ketones are tested to assess severity of acidosis and to monitor treatment response. Early detection of ketonuria is essential because ketoacidosis is a factor associated with intrauterine death.

Maternal ketonuria in women with post-term pregnancy is associated with a >twofold increase in the occurrence of oligohydramnios, and a significant increase in fetal heart rate decelerations (Onyeije 2001).

Further reading

Onyeije, C.I., Divon, M.Y., 2001. The impact of maternal ketonuria on fetal test results in the setting of postterm pregnancy. Am. J. Obstet. Gynecol. 184 (4), 713–718.

Kidney disease

Kidney disease can cause complications in pregnancy, pregnancy can cause complications in women with kidney disease and pregnancy can itself cause renal impairment.

Women with preexisting kidney disease should discuss the risks with their kidney specialist before trying to conceive. There is good evidence to suggest that women with very mild kidney disease (stages 1–2), normal blood pressure and little or no proteinuria can have a healthy pregnancy. In women with moderate to severe kidney disease (stages 3–5), the risk of complications is much greater, and for some women the risk to both the mother and baby are so high that pregnancy should be avoided.

In pregnancy, glomerular filtration rate increases up to 150% of the non-pregnant rate, and levels of urea and creatinine are decreased. Values which are considered normal in non-pregnant women may indicate decreased renal function in pregnancy. Creatinine >75 μmol/L and urea >4.5 mmol/L should prompt further investigation. Estimated glomerular filtration rate (eGFR) is not recommended in pregnancy. Glycosuria is common in pregnancy and does not necessarily indicate diabetes or impaired glucose tolerance. In the absence of infection, women with proteinuria greater than +1 on dipstick testing should have their level of proteinuria quantified (24-hour urine collection). Persistent proteinuria >500 mg/day before 20 weeks gestation should be referred promptly to a kidney specialist.

Asymptomatic urinary tract infection (UTI) and bacteriuria should be treated with antibiotics to reduce the risk of pyelonephritis, intrauterine growth restriction, fetal death and preterm labour.

Kidney disease can present for the first time during pregnancy, and women suspected to have kidney disease should be referred to a kidney specialist.

Further reading

Henderson, R., 2014. Renal disease in pregnancy. (Professional reference.) http://patient.info/doctor/renal-disease-in-pregnancy.

Medscape, 2015. Renal disease and pregnancy. http://emedicine.medscape.com/article/246123-overview.

National Kidney Foundation, 2016. Pregnancy and kidney disease. https://www.kidney.org/atoz/content/pregnancy.

Kleihauer test

A blood test used to measure the amount of fetal haemoglobin transferred from a fetus to the mother's bloodstream. It is performed on Rh-negative mothers to determine the dose of Anti-D immunoglobulin to inhibit formation of Rh antibodies in the mother and prevent Rh disease in future Rh-positive children. It is performed on an anticoagulated maternal blood sample within 2 hours of birth.

Klinefelter syndrome

Klinefelter syndrome is a chromosomal abnormality affecting around one in 600 newborn boys, in which the boy is born with an extra X chromosome (XXY). It is not usually diagnosed before the expected onset of puberty, although some boys will be born with undescended testicles. Males with Klinefelter syndrome may not produce sufficient testosterone to develop secondary male characteristics, and in adulthood, fertility may be affected because the testicles will produce little or no sperm.

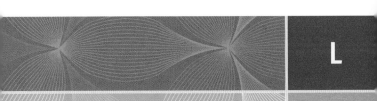

L

Laboratory results

The reference values for laboratory results are presented in Table 5.

Labour

Labour is the process of delivering the baby, the placenta, membranes and umbilical cord from the uterus via the vagina to the outside world. Regular uterine contractions, together with pressure from the descending, presenting part (the fetal head, or buttocks in a *breech* presentation), result in effacement and dilatation of the cervix to allow delivery of the baby.

Normal labour is spontaneous in onset between 37 and 42 weeks' gestation. The process of labour is described as three stages (see following).

Onset of labour

* Levels of maternal oestrogen rise sharply during the last weeks of pregnancy, overcoming the inhibiting effects of progesterone.
* Oestrogen stimulates the release of prostaglandins that help to soften the cervix.
* Uterine activity may result from mechanical stimulation of pressure from the presenting part of the fetus, well applied to the cervix.
* Contractions will often be accompanied or preceded by a blood-stained mucoid 'show', when the operculum, which formed the cervical plug during pregnancy, is lost as the cervix begins to dilate.

Table 5 **Laboratory reference values**

	Normal range (non-pregnant typical range)	Pregnant typical range	Normal range (neonates)
Haematology			
Haemoglobin (women)	11.5–16.5 g/dL	10.0–12.0 (≥10 in third trimester)	$17.0–21.0 \times 10^9$/L
Mean cell volume	76–96 mL		
Platelets	$150–400 \times 10^9$ L	Slight decrease in normal pregnancy	$150–450 \times 10^9$/L
White cells (total) Neutrophils Lymphocytes Eosinophils	$4–11 \times 10^9$ L 40%–75% 20%–45% 1%–6%	$9.0–15.0 \times 10^9$/L	$9–40 \times 10^9$/L
Fibrinogen	1.7–4.1 g/L	2.9–6.2 g/L (at term)	
Biochemistry			
Urea and electrolytes (U&E)			
Sodium	135–145 mmol/L		133–145 mmol/L
Potassium	3.5–5.3 mmol/L	Unchanged	3.5–6.0 mmol/L
Creatinine	50–100 μmol/L	75 μmol/L approx. is upper limit of normal	15–55 μmol/L
Urea	2–6.5 mmol/L	Usually ≤4.5 mmol/L	1.7–6.7 mmol/L
Uric acid	150–350 μmol/L		
Calcium	2.12–2.65 mmol/L		2.10–2.80 mmol/L
Albumin	30–48 mmol/L	25–35 mmol/L	
Proteins	60–80 g/L		
Liver function tests			
Bile acids	<9 μmol/L		
Bilirubin	<17 μmol/L		
Alanine transaminase (ALT)	6–40 IU/L	No change	≤40 IU/L
Aspartate transaminase (AST)	<50 IU/L		≤60 IU/L
Alkaline phosphatase	40–120 IU/L	Doubled by late pregnancy	
Cardiac enzymes			
Creatine kinase	25–195 IU/L		

Table 5 Laboratory reference values—cont'd

	Normal range (non-pregnant typical range)	Pregnant typical range	Normal range (neonates)
Lactate dehydrogenase (LDH)	70–150 IU/L		
Lipids			
Total cholesterol	<5 mmol/L (desired)[a]		
High density lipoprotein (HDL) cholesterol	>1.2 mmol/L (desired)		
Low density lipoprotein (LDL) cholesterol	<3 mmol/L (desired)[b]		
TC:HDL ratio	≤4.5 (desired)		
Triglycerides	0.5–1.9 mmol/L		
Other			
Albumin	30–48 g/L	25–35 g/L	25–45 g/L
Amylase	60–200 Somogyi unit/dL 70–300 IU/L (depending on method used)		
C-reactive protein (CRP)	<10 mg/L		
Blood glucose (fasting)	3.5–5.5 mmol/L		
T4 (total thyroxine)	70–140 mmol/L		
Thyroid stimulating hormone (TSH)	0.5–5 mIU/L		
Blood gases			
pH	7.35–7.45		
PaO_2	>10.6 kPa/ 75–100 mmHg		
$PaCo_2$	4.7–6 kPa/ 35–45 mmHg		
Base excess	±2 mmol/L		

N.B. Some ranges will vary between laboratories and this is only a guide. Check reference values with your local laboratory.
[a]<4 mmol/L in the presence of CHD, CKD, diabetes, stroke/TIA.
[b]<2 mmol/L in the presence of CHD, CKD, diabetes, stroke/TIA.

+ The membranes may also rupture: women should be advised to report this so the midwife can check that there are no changes in the fetal heart rate and that meconium is not present in the liquor.

Phases of the first stage of labour

The latent phase

+ Precedes the active first stage of labour
+ May last 6–8 hours in first time mothers
+ The cervix dilates from 0 cm to 3–4 cm
+ The cervical canal shortens from 3 cm to less than 0.5 cm

Active first stage

+ Begins when the cervix is 3–4 cm dilated
+ In the presence of rhythmic contractions, this stage is complete when the cervix is fully dilated (10 cm)
+ Usually completed within 6–12 hours

Transitional phase

+ The cervix expands from around 8 cm until it is fully dilated (or until the expulsive contractions during the second phase are felt by the woman).
+ There is often a brief lull in uterine activity at this time.

Second stage

The second phase of labour is the phase between full dilatation of the cervical os and the birth of the baby. Contractions become stronger and longer but may be less frequent. The membranes often rupture spontaneously (if they have not already done so). Fetal axis pressure increases flexion of the head, which results in smaller presenting diameters.

Contractions become expulsive as the fetus descends further into the vagina. Pressure from the presenting part stimulates nerve receptors in the pelvic floor and the woman experiences the urge to push. This reflex becomes increasingly compulsive and involuntary during each contraction. The mother's response is to employ her secondary powers of expulsion by contracting her abdominal muscles and diaphragm.

The fetal head becomes visible at the vulva, advancing with each contraction and receding between contractions until crowning takes place. The head is then born. The shoulders and body follow with the next contraction, accompanied by a gush of amniotic fluid and sometimes blood. The second stage culminates with the birth of the baby.

The time taken to complete the second stage of labour will vary considerably. Although some maternity units impose limits on its duration beyond which medical help should be called, these are not based on good evidence.

Third stage

During the third stage of labour, separation of the placenta and membranes occurs as the result of an interplay of mechanical and haemostatic factors. The time taken for the placenta to separate from the uterine wall can vary, but any period up to 1 hour may be considered to be within normal limits. Once separation has occurred, the uterus contracts strongly, contributing to haemostasis, and expelling the placenta and membranes into the vagina.

Uterotonic drugs such as ergometrine or oxytocin may be administered to stop the risk of bleeding or if it is deemed that there is a risk of excessive bleeding.

Further reading

National Institute for Health and Care Excellence, 2014. Intrapartum care for healthy women and babies. Clinical guideline CG190. https://www.nice.org.uk/guidance/cg190.

Royal College of Midwives, 2012. Evidence based guidelines for midwifery-led care in labour: latent phase. https://www.rcm.org.uk/sites/default/files/Latent%20Phase_1.pdf.

Royal College of Midwives, 2012. Evidence based guidelines for midwifery-led care in labour: second stage of labour. https://www.rcm.org.uk/sites/default/files/Second%20Stage%20of%20Labour.pdf.

Lactation

Lactation is the term for the production of milk by the breasts to nourish the baby from birth until it is weaned.

During pregnancy oestrogen and progesterone prepare the breast for lactation. Although colostrum is present from the 16th week of pregnancy, production of milk does not occur until after the birth, when placental hormone levels fall, allowing already high levels of prolactin to initiate milk production. Continued production of prolactin is caused by the baby feeding at the breast. Prolactin is involved in the suppression of ovulation and some women remain anovular until lactation ceases.

As lactation progresses, the prolactin response to suckling diminishes and milk removal becomes the driving force behind milk production.

Milk release—the 'let down' process—is under neuroendocrine control, and is stimulated by the release of oxytocin (see Oxytocin).

Milk production is largely independent of the mother's nutritional status and fluid intake and the practice of encouraging breastfeeding mothers to eat excessively should be abandoned.

> **Further reading**
>
> Medscape, 2015. Human milk and lactation. http://emedicine.
>   medscape.com/article/1835675-overview.

Løvset manoeuvre

The Løvset manoeuvre is used to deliver the shoulders in a breech presentation, when the arms are extended. The baby is held by the iliac crests, with thumbs over the sacrum and turned half a circle, keeping the back uppermost and applying downward traction at the same time, so that the arm that was posterior becomes anterior and can be delivered under the pubic arch. Delivery of the arm is assisted by placing one or two fingers on the upper part of the arm. Draw the arm down over the chest as the elbow is flexed, with the hand sweeping over the face. To deliver the second arm, the baby is rotated back half a circle, keeping the back uppermost and applying downward traction the second arm is delivered in the same way under the pubic arch.

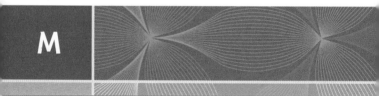

M

Mastitis

Mastitis means inflammation of the breast. In the majority of cases it is caused by milk stasis, not infection, although infection may supervene. Typically, one or more adjacent segments of the breast are inflamed and appear as a wedge-shaped area of redness and swelling. In some cases, flu-like symptoms, including shivering and/or rigors, may occur.

Acute inflammatory mastitis

This may occur during the early days of breastfeeding as a result of unresolved engorgement (milk stasis) or at any time when milk from one or more segments of the breast is not removed efficiently by the baby. It occurs most frequently in the breast opposite the mother's preferred side for holding her baby. It is important to continue feeding from the affected breast to avoid further milk stasis, which provides ideal conditions for pathogenic bacteria to replicate.

Infective mastitis

The main cause of superficial breast infection is damage to the epithelium, which allows bacteria to enter underlying tissues. This can result from incorrect attachment of the baby to the nipple. The mother will require help to improve her technique, as well as appropriate antibiotic therapy. Infection may also enter the breast via the milk ducts if milk stasis remains unresolved. In spite of antibiotic therapy, abscess formation may occur.

Breast abscess

A fluctuating swelling develops in a previously inflamed area. Pus may be discharged from the nipple. Simple needle aspiration may be effective or incision and drainage may be necessary. It may not be possible to feed from the affected breast for a few days but milk removal should be continued and breastfeeding should recommence as soon as practicable to reduce the chances of further abscess formation.

Further reading

Harding, M., 2015. Puerperal mastitis. (Professional reference.) http://patient.info/doctor/puerperal-mastitis.

Mauriceau–Smellie–Veit manoeuvre

The Mauriceau–Smellie–Veit manoeuvre (Fig. 20) is a manoeuvre to deliver the after-coming head in a breech, which involves jaw flexion and shoulder traction. The baby's body is laid across the practitioner's arm and the index fingers of one hand are placed on the malar bones of the baby's face, with the middle finger of the opposite hand applying pressure to the occiput to aid flexion. Traction is applied to draw the head out of the vagina and, when the sub-occipital region appears, the body is lifted to assist the head to pivot around the symphysis pubis. The speed of the birth must be controlled. Once the face is free, the airways may be cleared if required.

McRoberts manoeuvre

A manoeuvre to rotate the angle of the symphysis pubis superiorly and release the impaction of the anterior shoulder in shoulder dystocia. The woman brings her knees up to her chest.

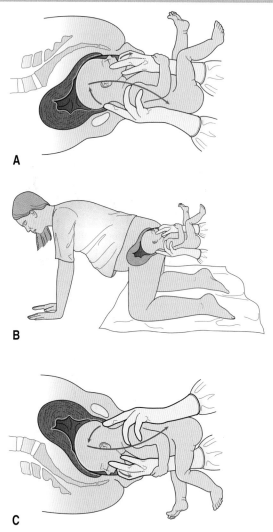

Fig. 20 Mauriceau-Smellie-Veit manoeuvre to assist the birth of the after-coming head in a breech presentation. (A) and (B) in the 'all fours' position and (C) in a semi-recumbent/sitting/adapted lithotomy position.

Meconium

Meconium is the stool of the fetus, formed before birth and composed of materials ingested in the uterus, including intestinal epithelial cells, lanugo, mucus, amniotic fluid, bile and water. Unlike later faeces it is viscous, sticky and tarlike and is usually very dark green in colour.

The presence of meconium in amniotic fluid in the second stage of labour is an indication of potential fetal compromise and experienced obstetric advice must be sought.

Most babies born through meconium stained liquor have not inhaled any particulate matter into the lower respiratory tract. However, if thick meconium is present and obstructing the airway, suction under direct vision should be performed. Meconium may also need to be aspirated from the trachea. This should only be carried out by a suitably trained medical professional.

Meconium aspiration syndrome

A baby can develop meconium aspiration syndrome if stimulated to breathe or gasp before or after birth when there is meconium in the airway that could be inhaled.

- The initial respiratory distress may be mild, moderate or severe, with a gradual deterioration over the first 12–24 hours in moderate or severe cases.
- The meconium becomes trapped in the airway and causes a ball-valve effect: air can be inhaled but is trapped behind the meconium blockage and cannot be exhaled.
- The accumulation of air can lead to rupture of the alveoli and cause the development of a pneumothorax.
- Where meconium is in contact with lung tissue, pneumonia may occur.
- Surfactant is broken down in the presence of meconium.

These factors combine with a previously hypoxic infant to produce a severe disease process. These babies will need full intensive care and ventilation to prevent further deterioration.

Further reading

MedlinePlus, 2013. Meconium aspiration syndrome. https://www.nlm.nih.gov/medlineplus/ency/article/001596.htm.

Vidyasagar, Bhat. Pathophysiology of meconium aspiration syndrome. BMJ Best Practice. http://bestpractice.bmj.com/best-practice/monograph/1185/basics/pathophysiology.html. (Log in or pay per view required.)

Membrane rupture

Rupture of the membranes

The optimum physiological time for the membranes to rupture spontaneously is at the end of the first stage of labour after the cervix becomes fully dilated and no longer supports the bag of forewaters.

+   The uterine contractions are also applying increasing force at this time.
+   Membranes may sometimes rupture days before labour begins or during the first stage.
+   If there are no other signs of labour but the history of ruptured membranes is convincing or obvious liquor is draining, then digital examination should be avoided owing to an increased risk of ascending infection.
+   If the diagnosis is not obvious, then one sterile speculum examination should be performed to try to visualize pooling of liquor in the posterior fornix; endocervical swabs may also be taken at this time.
+   The majority of women will labour spontaneously within 48 hours. After 48 hours an obstetrician may consider augmentation of labour.
+   Women with prelabour ruptured membranes should have their temperature recorded and be monitored for signs of fetal compromise associated with infection.
+   Occasionally, the membranes do not rupture, even in the second stage, and appear at the vulva as a bulging sac covering the fetal head as it is born; this is known as the 'caul'.

Sweeping or stripping of membrane

Sweeping the membranes can be an effective method of inducing labour in an uncomplicated pregnancy. During a vaginal examination, the clinician inserts a finger through the cervical os, and using a sweeping or circular movement, releases the fetal membranes from the lower uterine segment. The woman should be made aware that this procedure may cause some discomfort and bleeding.

Multiple pregnancy

The term multiple pregnancy describes the development of more than one fetus in the uterus at the same time (Fig. 21).

Twin pregnancy

Types of twin pregnancy

Twins will be either monozygotic (MZ) or dizygotic (DZ). In the UK, approximately two-thirds will be DZ and one-third MZ.

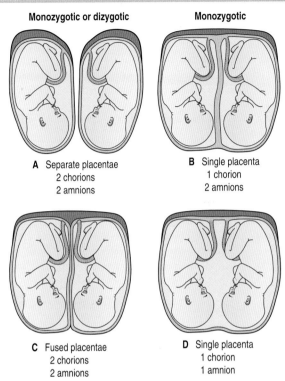

Monozygotic or dizygotic

A Separate placentae
2 chorions
2 amnions

Monozygotic

B Single placenta
1 chorion
2 amnions

C Fused placentae
2 chorions
2 amnions

D Single placenta
1 chorion
1 amnion

Fig. 21 **Multiple pregnancy.**

Superfecundation is the term used when twins are conceived from sperm from different men if a woman has had more than one partner during a menstrual cycle. It is not known how often this happens, but if suspected then paternity can be checked by DNA testing.

Superfetation is the term used for twins conceived as the result of two coital acts in different menstrual cycles. This is thought to be very rare.

Monozygosity and dizygosity
Monozygotic or uniovular twins
+ Also referred to as 'identical twins'
+ Develop from the fusion of one oocyte and one spermatozoon, which after fertilization splits into two

+ Are of the same sex and have the same genes, blood groups and physical features such as eye and hair colour, ear shapes and palm creases; may be of different sizes and sometimes have different personalities

Dizygotic or binovular twins

+ Also referred to as 'nonidentical twins'
+ Develop from two separate oocytes that are fertilized by two different spermatozoa
+ Are no more alike than any brother or sister and can be of the same or different sex

Diagnosis of twin pregnancy

This is usually through ultrasound examination. Diagnosis can be made as early as 6 weeks into the pregnancy, or later at the routine detailed structural scan between the 18th and 20th weeks. A family history of twins should alert the midwife to the possibility of a multiple pregnancy. Occasionally (1 in 12,000 live births), one fetus may die in the second trimester and become a fetus papyraceous, which becomes embedded in the surface of the placenta and expelled with the placenta at delivery.

Abdominal examination

Inspection

+ The size of the uterus may be larger than expected for the period of gestation, particularly after the 20th week. The uterus may look broad or round
+ Fetal movements may be seen over a wide area, although the findings are not diagnostic of twins
+ Fresh striae gravidarum may be apparent
+ Up to twice the amount of amniotic fluid is normal in a twin pregnancy but polyhydramnios is not an uncommon complication of a twin pregnancy, particularly with monochorionic twins

Palpation

+ The fundal height may be greater than expected for the period of gestation
+ The presence of two fetal poles (head or breech) in the fundus of the uterus may be noted; multiple fetal limbs may also be palpable
+ The head may be small in relation to the size of the uterus
+ Lateral palpation may reveal two fetal backs or limbs on both sides
+ Pelvic palpation may give findings similar to those on fundal palpation, although one fetus may lie behind the other and make detection difficult
+ Location of three poles in total is diagnostic of at least two fetuses

Auscultation

+ Hearing two fetal hearts is not diagnostic; however, if simultaneous comparison of the heart rates reveals a difference of at least 10 beats per minute, it may be assumed that two hearts are being heard

The pregnancy

A multiple pregnancy tends to be shorter than a single pregnancy. The average gestation for twins is 37 weeks, for triplets 34 weeks and for quadruplets 33 weeks.

Effects of pregnancy

Exacerbation of common disorders. More than one fetus and the higher levels of circulating hormones often exacerbate the common disorders of pregnancy. Sickness, nausea and heartburn may be more persistent and more troublesome than in a singleton pregnancy.

Anaemia. Iron deficiency and folic acid deficiency anaemias are common. Early growth and development of the uterus and its contents make greater demands on the maternal iron stores; in later pregnancy (after the 28th week) fetal demands may lead to anaemia. Routine prescription of iron and folic acid supplements is not necessary.

Polyhydramnios. This is particularly associated with monochorionic twins and with fetal abnormalities. Polyhydramnios will add to any discomfort that the woman is already experiencing. Acute polyhydramnios can lead to miscarriage or premature labour.

Pressure symptoms. Impaired venous return from the lower limbs increases the tendency to varicose veins and oedema of the legs. Backache is common and the increased uterine size may also lead to marked dyspnoea and to indigestion.

Other effects

There can be an increase in complications of pregnancy.

Antenatal screening

+ Nuchal translucency for Down syndrome is accurate only if performed between 11 and 13 weeks.
+ Serum screening is not usually performed in multiple pregnancy, as results are too complex to interpret.
+ Chorionic villus sampling (CVS) is not usually recommended in multiple pregnancy, as loss rates are high.

- Amniocentesis can be performed in twin pregnancies, usually between 15 and 20 weeks. It should be performed in a specialist fetal medicine unit. Most obstetricians prefer to do a dual needle insertion so there is no chance of contamination between the two sacs.
- Chorionicity should be determined in the first trimester.
- All MZ twins should have echocardiography performed at approximately 20 weeks' gestation, as there is a much higher risk of cardiac anomalies in these babies.

Ultrasound examination

- Monochorionic twin pregnancies should be scanned every 2 weeks from diagnosis to check for discordant fetal growth and signs of twin-to-twin transfusion syndrome (TTTS).
- Dichorionic twin pregnancies should be scanned at 20 weeks for anomalies, and then usually every 4 weeks.

Antenatal preparation

Early diagnosis of a twin pregnancy and of chorionicity is extremely important in order to support and advise the parents.

Preparation for breastfeeding

Mothers should be advised not only that it is possible to breastfeed two, and in some cases three, babies, but also that, nutritionally, this is the best way for her to feed her babies.

Labour and birth
Onset of labour

The higher the number of fetuses the mother is carrying, the earlier the labour is likely to start. Term for twins is usually considered to be 37 weeks rather than 40, and approximately 30% of twins are born preterm. In addition to being preterm the babies may be small for gestational age and therefore prone to the associated complications of both conditions. If spontaneous labour begins very early the mother may be given drugs to inhibit uterine activity. Known causes of preterm labour, for example urinary tract infection, should be treated with antibiotics.

It is very unusual for a twin pregnancy to last more than 40 weeks; many obstetricians advise induction of labour at 38 weeks. If the first twin is in a cephalic presentation, labour is usually allowed to continue normally to a vaginal birth, but if the first twin is presenting in any other way, an elective caesarean section is usually recommended.

Management of labour

Induction of labour usually occurs around 38 weeks' gestation. The presence of complications such as pregnancy-induced hypertension, intrauterine growth restriction or TTTS may be reasons for earlier induction.

The majority will go into labour spontaneously. There is an increased incidence of dysfunctional labour in twin pregnancies, possibly because of overdistension of the uterus.

+ Continuous fetal heart monitoring of both babies is advocated. This can be achieved with two external transducers, or once the membranes are ruptured, with a scalp electrode on the presenting twin and an external transducer on the second.
+ If a 'twin monitor' is available, both heartbeats can be monitored simultaneously to give a more reliable reading. Uterine activity will also need to be monitored.
+ If cardiotocography (CTG) is not available, use of Doppler fetal monitoring may give more accurate recordings of the fetal heart rates than a fetal stethoscope. If the latter has to be used, two people must auscultate simultaneously so that fetal heart rates are counted over the same minute.

Mobilization or the adoption of whichever position the mother finds most comfortable should be encouraged. A foam rubber wedge under the side of the mattress will help to prevent supine hypotensive syndrome by giving a lateral tilt. A birthing chair or a reclining chair may be more comfortable than a delivery bed.

Regional epidural block provides excellent analgesia and, if necessary, allows easier instrumental deliveries and also manipulation of the second twin. The use of inhalation analgesia may be helpful, either before the epidural is in situ or during the second stage if the effect of the epidural is wearing off.

+ If fetal compromise occurs during labour, delivery will need to be expedited, usually by caesarean section. Action may also need to be taken if the mother's condition gives cause for concern.
+ If uterine activity is poor, the use of intravenous oxytocin may be required once the membranes have been ruptured.
+ If the babies are expected to be premature and of low birth weight or known to have any other problems, the neonatal unit must be informed.

Management of the births

The second stage of labour may be confirmed by a vaginal examination. The obstetrician, paediatric team and anaesthetist should be present for the births because of the risk of complications.

+ If epidural analgesia has been used, it may be 'topped up'.
+ The possibility of emergency caesarean section is ever-present and the operating theatre should be ready to receive the mother at short notice.
+ Monitoring of both fetal hearts should continue.
+ Provided that the first twin is presenting by the vertex, the birth can be expected to proceed normally.
+ When the first twin is born, the time of birth and the sex are noted, and the baby and cord must be labelled as 'twin 1' immediately.
+ The baby may be put to the breast because suckling stimulates uterine contractions.
+ If the first baby requires active resuscitation, the paediatric team will take over.
+ After the birth of the first twin, abdominal palpation is carried out to ascertain the lie, presentation and position of the second twin and to auscultate the fetal heart:
    + If the lie is not longitudinal, an attempt may be made to correct it by external cephalic version.
    + If it is longitudinal, a vaginal examination is made to confirm the presentation.
    + If the presenting part is not engaged, it should be guided into the pelvis by fundal pressure before the second sac of membranes is ruptured.
+ The fetal heart should be auscultated again once the membranes are ruptured.
+ If uterine activity does not recommence, intravenous oxytocin may be used to stimulate it.
+ When the presenting part becomes visible, the mother should be encouraged to push with contractions to birth the second twin.
+ The reduced size of the placental site following the birth of the first twin means that the second fetus may be somewhat deprived of oxygen.
+ The birth of the second twin should be completed within 45 minutes of the first twin as long as there are no signs of fetal distress in the second twin; if there are, the birth must be expedited and the second twin may need to be delivered by caesarean section.
+ A uterotonic drug is usually given intramuscularly or intravenously, depending on local policy, after the birth of the anterior shoulder.
+ Record the time of birth and sex of this baby, and label the baby and cord as 'twin 2'.
+ The risk of asphyxia is greater for the second twin. The baby may need to be transferred to the neonatal unit, but should be shown to the mother prior to transfer.

- Once the uterotonic drug has taken effect, controlled cord traction is applied to both cords simultaneously and the placentae should be delivered without delay. Emptying the uterus enables bleeding to be controlled and postpartum haemorrhage (PPH) prevented. An infusion of 40 IU of Syntocinon in 500 mL of normal saline should be prepared for prophylactic use in the management of PPH.
- The placenta(e) should be examined and the number of amniotic sacs, chorions and placentae noted. Pathological examination of placentae and membranes may be needed to confirm chorionicity.

Complications associated with multiple pregnancy

The high perinatal mortality associated with twinning is largely due to complications of pregnancy, such as the premature onset of labour, intrauterine growth restriction and complications of delivery.

Polyhydramnios

Acute polyhydramnios may occur as early as 18–20 weeks. It may be associated with fetal abnormality but it is more likely to be due to TTTS.

Twin-to-twin transfusion syndrome

Also known as fetofetal transfusion syndrome (FFTS), this can be acute or chronic. The acute form usually occurs during labour and is the result of a blood transfusion from one fetus (donor) to the other (recipient) through vascular anastomosis in a monochorionic placenta. Both fetuses may die of cardiac failure if not treated immediately.

Chronic FFTS can occur in up to 35% of monochorionic twin pregnancies and accounts for 15%–17% of perinatal mortality in twins. The placenta transfuses blood from one twin fetus to the other. Fetal and/or neonatal mortality is high but some infants may be saved by early diagnosis and prenatal treatment. Selective fetocide is sometimes considered.

Fetal abnormality

This is particularly associated with MZ twins.

Conjoined twins. This extremely rare malformation of MZ twinning results from the incomplete division of the fertilized oocyte. Delivery has to be by caesarean section. Separation of the babies is sometimes possible and will depend on how they are joined and which internal organs are involved.

Acardiac twins (twin reversed arterial perfusion [TRAP]). One twin presents without a well-defined cardiac structure and is kept alive through placental anastomoses to the circulatory system of the viable fetus.

Fetus-in-fetu (endoparasite). Parts of one fetus may be lodged within another fetus; this can happen only in MZ twins.

Malpresentations

The fetuses can restrict each other's movements, which may result in malpresentations, particularly of the second twin. After the birth of the first twin, the presentation of the second twin may change.

Premature rupture of the membranes. Malpresentations due to poly-hydramnios may predispose to preterm rupture of the membranes.

Prolapse of the cord. This is associated with malpresentations and poly-hydramnios and is more likely if there is a poorly fitting presenting part. The second twin is particularly at risk.

Prolonged labour. Malpresentations are a poor stimulus to good uterine action and a distended uterus is likely to lead to poor uterine activity and consequently prolonged labour.

Monoamniotic twins. Monoamniotic twins risk cord entanglement with occlusion of the blood supply to one or both fetuses. Delivery is usually at around 32–34 weeks and by caesarean section.

Locked twins. This is a rare but serious complication. There are two types: one occurs when the first twin presents by the breech and the second by the vertex, the other when both are vertex presentations. In both instances the head of the second twin prevents the continued descent of the first.

Delay in the birth of the second twin

After delivery of the first twin, uterine activity should recommence within 5 minutes. Birth of the second twin is usually completed within 45 minutes of the first birth. In the past the birth interval was limited to 30 minutes in an attempt to minimize complications. With the introduction of fetal heart rate monitoring the interval time between babies is not so crucial as long as the fetal condition is monitored. Poor uterine action as a result of malpresentation may be the cause of delay. The risks of delay are:

+ intrauterine hypoxia;
+ birth asphyxia following premature separation of the placenta; and
+ sepsis as a result of ascending infection from the first umbilical cord, which lies outside the vulva.

After the birth of the first twin the lower uterine segment begins to reform and the cervical canal may have to dilate fully again.

The midwife may need to 'rub up' a contraction and to put the first twin to the mother's breast to stimulate uterine activity.

* If there appears to be an obstruction, a caesarean section may be necessary.
* If there is no obstruction, oxytocin infusion may be commenced or forceps delivery considered.

Premature expulsion of the placenta

The placenta may be expelled before delivery of the second twin.

* In dichorionic twins with separate placentae, one placenta may be delivered separately.
* In monochorionic twins, the shared placenta may be expelled. The risks of severe asphyxia and death of the second twin are then very high.
* Haemorrhage is also likely if one twin is retained in utero, as this prevents adequate retraction of the placental site.

Postpartum haemorrhage

Poor uterine tone as a result of over distension or hypotonic activity is likely to lead to postpartum haemorrhage.

Undiagnosed twins

The possibility of an unexpected undiagnosed second baby should be considered if the uterus appears larger than expected after the birth of the first baby or if the baby is surprisingly smaller than expected. If a uterotonic drug has been given after the birth of the anterior shoulder of the first baby, the second baby is in great danger and delivery should be expedited. He or she will require active resuscitation because of severe asphyxia.

Postnatal period
Care of the babies

Immediate care at delivery is the same as for a single baby. Identification of the infants should be clear and the parents should be given the opportunity to check the identity bracelets and cuddle their babies.

Nutrition

Both babies may be breastfed, either simultaneously or separately. The mother may choose to feed artificially.

* If the babies are small for gestational age or preterm, the pae-diatrician may recommend that the babies be 'topped up' after a

breastfeed. Expressed breast milk is the best form of nutrition for these babies.

+ If the babies are not able to suck adequately at the breast, then the mother should be encouraged to express her milk regularly for her babies.

+ If she does not have sufficient milk for them, milk from a human milk bank can be used, which is much better for preterm babies than formula milk.

The more stimulation the breasts are given, the more plentiful is the milk supply.

Care of the mother

Involution of the uterus will be slower because of its increased bulk. 'Afterpains' may be troublesome and analgesia should be offered.

A good diet is essential, and if the mother is breastfeeding, she requires a high-protein, high-calorie diet.

Once the mother is at home she must be encouraged to rest and eat a well-balanced diet.

The incidence of postnatal depression has been shown to be significantly higher in twin mothers.

Triplets and higher-order births

A woman expecting three or more babies is at risk of all the same complications as one expecting twins, but more so. She is more likely to have a period in hospital resting before the babies are born and they will almost certainly be delivered prematurely. Perinatal mortality rates are higher for triplets than twins and the incidence of cerebral palsy is also increased.

The mode of delivery for triplets or more babies is usually by caesarean section. It is essential that the paediatric team be present. The special dangers associated with these births are:

+ asphyxia
+ intracranial injury
+ perinatal death

Perinatal mortality and long-term morbidity are both more common among multiple births than singletons. The perinatal mortality rate for twins is about four times that of singletons, and that of triplets 12 times higher.

Embryo reduction

This is the reduction of an apparently healthy higher-order multiple pregnancy down to two or even one embryo so the chances of survival are much higher. The procedure may be offered to parents who have conceived triplets or more.

The procedure is usually carried out between the 10th and 12th weeks of the pregnancy. Various techniques may be used, involving the insertion of a needle under ultrasound guidance either via the vagina or, more commonly, through the abdominal wall into the fetal thorax. Potassium chloride is usually used, although some doctors prefer saline. All embryos remain in the uterus until birth.

Selective fetocide

This may be offered to parents with a multiple pregnancy when one of the babies has a serious abnormality. The affected fetus is injected as described in embryo reduction, so allowing the healthy fetus to grow and develop normally.

Further reading

National Institute for Health and Care Excellence, 2011. Multiple pregnancy: antenatal care for twin and triplet pregnancies. Clinical guideline 129. https://www.nice.org.uk/guidance/CG129.

Royal College of Obstetricians and Gynaecologists, 2008. Management of monochorionic twin pregnancy. Green-top guideline no. 51. https://www.rcog.org.uk/en/guidelines-research-services/guidelines/gtg51/.

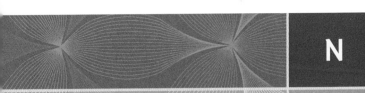

N

Nausea

Nausea and vomiting are common symptoms in early pregnancy, usually starting between 4 and 10 weeks' gestation and resolving before 20 weeks. Hyperemesis gravidarum is defined as persistent pregnancy-related vomiting associated with weight loss of >5% of total body mass and ketosis. Affecting 0.3%–3% of all pregnant women, this condition is associated with dehydration, electrolyte imbalance and thiamine deficiency (see Hyperemesis gravidarum).

The impact of nausea and vomiting on the woman and her daily life should not be underestimated. The midwife should enquire of all women attending for early antenatal care whether they are experiencing nausea or vomiting. If vomiting is mild to moderate, and not causing signs of dehydration, then usually reassurance and advice will be all that is necessary.

Simple measures include:
- taking small, carbohydrate meals
- avoiding large volume drinks, especially milk and carbonated drinks
- raising the head of the bed if reflux is a problem

Antiemetic therapy is reserved for those women who do not settle on supportive measures, or who persistently relapse. The use of antiemetics in pregnancy received widespread publicity when links were found between thalidomide and severe malformations of children born to mothers who had taken the drug for morning sickness. Currently antihistamines are the recommended first line treatment for nausea and vomiting in pregnancy—no antiemetic is approved for this indication.

Ginger is a well-known traditional herb remedy for sickness and there is considerable research to demonstrate that it is an effective antiemetic. However, it is not suitable for all women and may exacerbate nausea and cause heartburn. Ginger biscuits should not be advised as any temporary improvement is attributable to their sugar content, and they contain insufficient ginger to have any real therapeutic effect.

There is no evidence for the effectiveness of homeopathic remedies. The use of travel sickness wristbands may be useful for some women, and acupuncture can also be effective.

Nausea in labour

Opiate drugs, including pethidine, diamorphine or meptazinol, are commonly used for pain relief in labour but side effects include nausea, vomiting and drowsiness in the mother, and depression of the baby's respiratory centre at birth. An antiemetic agent is sometimes given at the same time to reduce nausea.

Needlestick/sharps injury

A skin puncture caused by a hypodermic needle or sharp or broken item of equipment (e.g., scalpel, mounted needle, broken glassware, etc.). A needlestick injury is of concern because of the risk of transmission of blood-borne viruses (e.g., hepatitis B [HBV], hepatitis C [HCV], human immunodeficiency virus [HIV]). The most common cause in healthcare professionals is attempted resheathing of needles.

If the sharp was used or dirty:

+ encourage wound to bleed, to expel contaminants
+ wash with soap and warm water. Do not scrub. Do not use antiseptics
+ dry and apply waterproof plaster
+ report to practice manager/senior partner immediately
+ assess risk—contact occupational health or local consultant in communicable disease control/consultant microbiologist/virologist or genitourinary medicine or A&E
+ complete accident form

See *Immunization Against Infectious Disease (The Green Book)* for prophylaxis and procedure where there is substantial risk of blood-borne infection (HIV or hepatitis), also for primary and reinforcing immunization.

Hepatitis B prophylaxis

HBV immunoglobulin (HBIG) confers passive immunity and gives immediate but temporary protection after accidental inoculation or contamination with HBV-infected blood. HBIG is recommended only in high-risk situations or a known nonresponder to vaccine. Should ideally be given within 48 hours of exposure, but can be considered at up to 1 week. An HBV vaccination course confers active immunity. If an unprotected individual is at high risk of infection, the vaccine can be given at the same time as HBIG.

Further reading

Bandolier. Needlestick injuries. http://www.bandolier.org.uk/booth/booths/needle.html.

Health and Safety Executive, 2016. Sharps injuries. http://www.hse.gov.uk/healthservices/needlesticks/.

Public Health England, 2014. Eye of the needle: United Kingdom surveillance of significant occupational exposure to bloodborne viruses in healthcare workers. https://www.gov.uk/government/uploads/system/uploads/attachment_data/file/385300/EoN_2014_-_FINAL_CT_3_sig_occ.pdf.

Public Health England. Immunisation Against Infectious Disease (The Green Book). https://www.gov.uk/government/collections/immunisation-against-infectious-disease-the-green-book.

Neonatal intensive care unit See Neonatal specialist care.

Neonatal infections

Newborns can acquire infections via a number of routes—from the placenta (transplacental infection), from amniotic fluid, from their passage through the birth canal, and from carers' hands, contaminated objects or droplet infection after birth.

Newborns are immunodeficient and prone to a higher incidence of infection. Preterm babies are even more vulnerable, as they have less well-developed defence mechanisms at birth (transfer of immunoglobulin G occurs after 32 weeks' gestation). They are also more likely to experience invasive procedures.

At birth the baby has some immune protection from the mother, from maternal antibodies developed in response to exposure to antigens.

Breastfeeding increases the baby's immune protection through the transmission of immunoglobulin A in breast milk. During the early weeks of life, the baby also has deficiencies in both the quantity and quality of neutrophils.

Individual risk factors for infection

- Maternal history of prolonged rupture of membranes
- Chorioamnionitis
- Pyrexia during birth
- Offensive amniotic fluid

The overall aim of management of neonatal infections is to provide prompt and effective treatment that reduces the risk of sepsis. Good management includes:

- caring for the baby in a thermoneutral environment and observing for temperature instability
- good hydration and correction of electrolyte imbalance, with demand feeding if possible, and intravenous fluids if required

Some specific neonatal infections are described below.

Group B streptococcus

The leading cause of serious neonatal infection in the UK is Group B streptococcus (GBS). Early onset (when symptoms develop within the first 5 days of life) suggests that the infection started in utero. In the USA, pregnant women are screened in the third trimester for GBS and are treated prophylactically with intrapartum penicillin if identified as high risk. Routine screening is not offered in the UK.

Syphilis

World Health Organization figures estimate that maternal syphilis affects 1 million pregnancies each year, with 460,000 resulting in abortion or perinatal death. In the UK, antenatal screening for syphilis is routine and the incidence of infectious syphilis is low. Vertical transmission may occur at any time during pregnancy in untreated early syphilis and the rate of vertical transmission in untreated women is 70%–100% for primary syphilis, but the risk of transmission diminishes as maternal syphilis advances.

The UK prevalence of congenital syphilis is very low, but is associated with serious neurological, developmental and musculoskeletal sequelae; the prognosis is considered poor if symptoms present in the first few weeks of life. Signs in symptomatic infants may be subtle and nonspecific, but characteristically include prematurity, low birthweight, hepatomegaly with or without splenomegaly and failure to thrive. Treatment is usually with penicillin.

Herpes simplex virus

Neonatal herpes is a severe systemic viral infection with high morbidity and mortality. The incidence in the UK is about 1.65 in 100,000 births and can be caused by either herpes simplex virus 1 (HSV-1) or herpes simplex virus 2 (HSV-2). Women who have had herpes prior to pregnancy will have developed antibodies to the virus, and the fetus will have passive immunity. The greatest risk to the fetus is therefore if the woman acquires a primary infection in late pregnancy. Congenital HSV infection can cause severe congenital abnormalities. About 70% of cases of neonatal HSV are caused by HSV-2 and result from contact with maternal genital secretions during delivery. Neonatal herpes can also be acquired from an ascending infection following rupture of the membranes.

Human immunodeficiency virus

As the incidence of human immunodeficiency virus (HIV) infection in women increases, so does the problem of vertical transmission. Worldwide, millions of children are infected, primarily through mother-to-child transmission during pregnancy or breastfeeding.

HIV-positive women should be offered an elective caesarean section as this is an effective way of reducing vertical transmission among women not taking antiretroviral drugs. In a woman with a low viral load, it is unclear whether caesarean section is more or less effective than vaginal birth.

Breastfeeding contributes significantly to vertical transmission of HIV and should be avoided if possible.

See also HIV, Ophthalmia neonatorum, Rubella, Toxoplasmosis, and Varicella zoster.

Further reading

National Institute for Health and Care Excellence (NICE), 2014. Neonatal infection. Quality standard 75. https://www.nice.org.uk/guidance/qs75.

NICE, 2012. Neonatal infection (early onset): antibiotics for prevention and treatment. Clinical guideline 149. https://www.nice.org.uk/guidance/cg149.

Neonatal specialist care

As a result of increasing rates of fertility and availability of assisted conception, increasing numbers of babies require specialist neonatal care each year. In England (2007–2008) one in ten babies born alive received specialist neonatal care. In particular, babies born preterm require highly specialized care in units where multidisciplinary teams can ensure they receive the best possible, technologically advanced care, and that the needs of their families are also met.

Parents of babies receiving specialist neonatal care should be encouraged to be involved in planning and providing care for their baby, and regular communication with clinical staff should occur throughout. Mothers should be supported to start and continue breastfeeding, including being supported to express milk.

Further reading

BLISS. About neonatal care. http://www.bliss.org.uk/about-neonatal-care.

National Institute for Health and Care Excellence, 2010. Neonatal specialist care. Quality standard QS4. https://www.nice.org.uk/guidance/qs4.

Neonatal screening

Babies are screened for inborn errors of metabolism and endocrine disorders, which are detected by means of a blood test, e.g., the Guthrie test.[a] This is taken on day 4–6 after birth for the detection of phenylketonuria,

---

[a]Blood is obtained from a heel prick made with a stilette on the lateral aspect of the heel (to avoid nerves and blood vessels) and dripped on to circles on an absorbent card, onto which full details of the baby's identity and history have been entered.

hypothyroidism, cystic fibrosis, sickle cell disease, medium-chain acyl-CoA dehydrogenase deficiency (MCADD), maple syrup urine, homocystinuria, glutaric acidaemia type 1 and isovalaeric acidaemia. Some centres also test routinely for galactosaemia, a rare inherited disease but among the most common disorders of carbohydrate metabolism; galactosaemia can be a life-threatening condition in the neonatal period.

Neural tube defects

Neural tube defects are birth defects of the brain, spine or spinal cord. They happen in the first month of pregnancy, often before the woman is aware that she is pregnant.

The most common such defects are spina bifida, in which the spinal column does not close completely, and anencephaly, in which the brain and cranium fail to develop. Most babies with anencephaly are either stillborn or die shortly after birth.

Most cases of neural tube defect can be prevented by ensuring adequate levels of folic acid.

Neural tube defect screening

Alpha fetoprotein (AFP) is present in fetal serum and amniotic fluid by 6 weeks' gestation. When the fetus has an open neural tube defect, AFP can escape in increased amounts, causing levels to be raised in maternal serum. A blood sample from the mother at 15–18 weeks has a detection rate of 98% but this test has largely been superseded by the use of ultrasound to diagnose a range of neural tube defects.

Nosocomial infections See Healthcare-acquired infections.

Nuchal translucency

The measurement of nuchal translucency (NT) at 10–14 weeks' gestation can provide information about the developing fetus. Increased NT is associated with chromosomal abnormalities, structural and genetic disorders. This information can be used in combination with maternal age and biochemical markers to assess the risk of Down syndrome. In general, mothers appreciate the opportunity for early information so that they can consider the option of termination before they are visibly pregnant and can feel the baby's movements. However, this can also be a disadvantage in that parents are faced with a decision about whether to terminate a pregnancy that may be destined to miscarry naturally. Approximately 40% of affected fetuses die between 12 weeks' gestation and term.

Nuchal fold measurement

Nuchal fold >5 mm at 20 weeks' gestation is a marker of chromosomal abnormality. After 14 weeks' gestation, nuchal translucency can no longer be visualized and the nuchal fold is measured instead. A thick nuchal fold is often considered to be the most sensitive and most specific second trimester marker for Down syndrome.

Nipples, anatomical variation

Long nipples can lead to poor feeding because the baby is able to latch on to the nipple without drawing breast tissue into his or her mouth. The mother may need to be shown how to help the baby draw in a sufficient portion of the breast.

Short nipples should not cause any problems as the baby has to form a teat from both the breast and nipple. The mother should be reassured.

Abnormally large nipples. If the baby is small, his/her mouth may not be able to get beyond the nipple and onto the breast. Lactation could be initiated by expressing. As the baby grows and the breast and nipple become more protractile, breastfeeding may become possible

Inverted and flat nipples. If the nipple is deeply inverted it *may* be necessary to initiate lactation by expressing. Attempts to attach the baby to the breast are delayed until lactation is established and the breasts have become soft and breast tissue is more protractile.

Nipples, sore

Sore and damaged nipples are almost always caused by trauma from the hard palate of the baby's mouth and tongue, resulting from incorrect attachment to the breast. Correcting this will provide immediate relief from pain and allow rapid healing to take place. Resting the nipple is not advised as, although this enables healing to take place, it may make continuation of lactation more difficult.

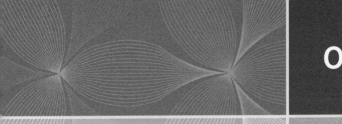

Obesity

Obesity is a growing concern in much of Europe, including the UK. Worldwide, 39% of adults aged 18 years and over were overweight. Obesity is defined as a body mass index (BMI) >30 kg/m^2. It is estimated that in the UK, approximately 1 in 20 women are obese during pregnancy.

Obesity in pregnancy is associated with a range of problems, including delivery complications and poor fetal outcomes. Obesity increases the risk of gestational diabetes, hypertension, preeclampsia, uncertain fetal position, urinary tract infections, postpartum haemorrhage and thromboembolic events. Women who are obese are more likely to require a caesarean section, and their babies are more like to be large or, ironically, small for gestational age.

Ideally, women will attempt to achieve a normal BMI (18.5–24.9 kg/m^2) before becoming pregnant. However, if overweight or obese when their pregnancy is confirmed they should be given the opportunity to discuss diet and other lifestyle factors from early in pregnancy and at regular intervals thereafter. Routine weighing is not recommended.

Further reading

Centre for Maternal and Child Enquiries, 2010. Maternal obesity in the UK: findings from a national project. http://www.publichealth.hscni.net/sites/default/files/Maternal%20Obesity%20in%20the%20UK.pdf.

World Health Organization, 2016. Obesity and overweight. http://www.who.int/mediacentre/factsheets/fs311/en/.

Obstetric cholestasis

Obstetric cholestasis (OC) or intrahepatic cholestasis of pregnancy (ICP) is a liver disorder that occurs in around one in 140 pregnancies (0.7%) in the UK, where the normal flow of bile out of the liver is reduced. Chemicals in the bile called bile salts (also often referred to as bile acids) can then build up and 'leak' into the bloodstream. This causes affected women to have increased levels of bile salts in their blood.

The condition is also characterized by itching, known as pruritus, which generally appears in the last 3 months of pregnancy (though it can appear sooner). It is of variable severity and can be extremely distressing for the mother. Both the raised bile salts and pruritus completely disappear soon after the birth and generally do not appear to cause long-term health problems for mothers.

There can be an increased risk of preterm delivery (both spontaneous and induced) and fetal distress. Some case studies have also reported stillbirth occurring near the end of pregnancy in women with the condition, therefore it is essential that the condition is recognized and treated in time.

At present, most maternity units in the UK managing women with OC/ICP pregnancies deliver babies early, at around 37 or 38 weeks. This is done because it is thought that it may help prevent the possibility of stillbirth. There have been no reports of any harmful effects to babies from OC/ICP pregnancies once they have been delivered. The clinical importance of OC/ICP is the potential risks to the fetus, including spontaneous preterm birth, iatrogenic preterm birth and fetal death.

OC/ICP is more common in multiple pregnancies, and is more common in women of Indian or Pakistani origin, affecting around 1 in 70 to 1 in 80 pregnancies (1.2%–1.5%). In South America and other countries such as Scandinavia, the number of women affected is higher still. Women with hepatitis C are at increased risk.

Itching is often the only symptom. It usually begins on the arms, legs, hands and soles of the feet, but can occur on other parts of the body. It is usually worse at night, leading to sleeplessness and exhaustion. Itching can be intense, and women can scratch themselves until they make themselves bleed. Some women will develop jaundice but most do not.

Diagnosis is made on the basis of symptoms and history and liver function tests, which will reveal raised levels of the liver enzymes alanine aminotransferase (ALT) and aspartate aminotransferase (AST). Sometimes gamma-glutamyl transferase (GGT) will also be raised. The most specific test involves measuring serum bile acids: levels greater than 14 µmol/L (10 µmol/L in a fasting blood sample) are considered raised.

Further reading

British Liver Trust, 2011. Obstetric cholestasis/intrahepatic cholestasis of pregnancy (ICP). http://www.britishlivertrust.org.uk/liver-information/liver-conditions/obstetric-cholestasis/.

Further reading—cont'd

National Institute for Health and Care Excellence, 2015. Clinical knowledge summaries. Itch in pregnancy. http://cks.nice.org.uk/itch-in-pregnancy.

Royal College of Obstetricians and Gynaecologists, 2011. Obstetric cholestasis. Green-top guideline no. 43. https://www.rcog.org.uk/en/guidelines-research-services/guidelines/gtg43/.

Obstructed labour

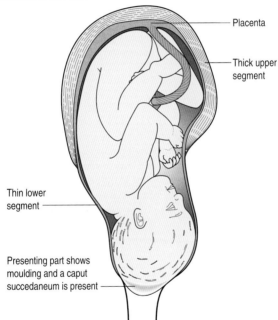

Fig. 22 **Obstructed labour.**

Labour is obstructed when there is no advance of the presenting part despite strong uterine contractions (Fig. 22). The obstruction usually occurs at the pelvic brim but may occur at the outlet.

Causes

+ Cephalopelvic disproportion
+ Deep transverse arrest

- Malpresentation (e.g., shoulder or brow presentation, or in persistent mentoposterior position)
- Pelvic mass (e.g., fibroids, ovarian or pelvic tumours)
- Fetal abnormalities

If obstructed labour is recognized in the first stage of labour, delivery should be by caesarean section.

Further reading

Royal College of Obstetricians and Gynaecologists, 2012. Shoulder dystocia. Green-top guideline no. 42. https://www.rcog.org.uk/en/guidelines-research-services/guidelines/gtg42/.

World Health Organization. Managing prolonged and obstructed labour. Midwifery education module 3. http://www.who.int/maternal_child_adolescent/documents/3_9241546662/en/.

Occipitoposterior positions

Occipitoposterior positions (Figs 23 and 24) are the most common type of malposition of the occiput and occur in approximately 10% of labours. A persistent occipitoposterior position results from a failure of internal rotation prior to delivery. The vertex is presenting but the occiput lies in the posterior rather than anterior part of the pelvis. As a result, the fetal head is deflexed and larger diameters of the fetal skull present. Labour

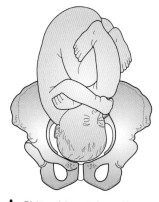 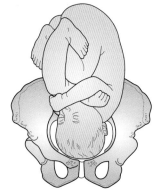

A Right occipitoposterior position   **B** Left occipitoposterior position

Fig. 23 Occipitoposterior positions.

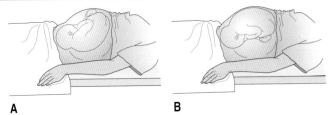

A   **B**

Fig. 24 Comparison of abdominal contour in (A) posterior and (B) anterior positions of the occiput.

with a fetus in an occipitoposterior position may be long and painful, and there is an increased risk of operative delivery.

> **Further reading**
>
> Royal College of Midwives, 2012. Evidence based guidelines for midwifery-led care in labour: persistent lateral and posterior fetal positions at the onset of labour. https://www.rcm.org.uk/sites/default/files/Persistent%20Lateral%20and%20Posterior%20Fetal%20Positions%20%20at%20the%20Onset%20of%20Labour.pdf.

Oedema

Oedema is defined as the retention of fluid in body tissues. It can occur in one part of the body, for example as the result of an injury, or it can be more general.

In pregnancy, oedema is unlikely to be observed at the initial assessment but may occur as the pregnancy progresses. Physiological oedema is often associated with daily activities or hot weather. Later in pregnancy the midwife should observe the woman for oedema and ask her about symptoms.

In multiple pregnancies, impaired venous return from the lower limbs increases the tendency to varicose veins and oedema.

Sudden appearance of severe, widespread oedema is suggestive of preeclampsia or some underlying pathology and further investigations are necessary.

Oligohydramnios

Oligohydramnios is an abnormally small amount of amniotic fluid. At term it may be 300–500 mL or even less. When diagnosed in the first half of pregnancy the condition is often found to be associated with renal agenesis (absence of kidneys) or Potter syndrome, in which the baby also has pulmonary hypoplasia. At any stage of pregnancy, it may be due to fetal abnormality or premature rupture of membranes where amniotic fluid fails to reaccumulate.

The lack of amniotic fluid reduces the intrauterine space and over time will cause compression deformities.

Diagnosis is with ultrasound examination to differentiate between oligohydramnios and intrauterine growth restriction.

Management

If the ultrasound demonstrates renal agenesis, the baby will not survive. Liquor volume will also be estimated from the scan; if renal agenesis is not present, further investigations will include careful placental function tests. Management may involve the following:

- Prophylactic amnioinfusion with normal saline, Ringer lactate or 5% glucose may be performed to prevent compression deformities and hypoplastic lung disease, and to prolong the pregnancy.
- Labour may occur spontaneously or be induced because of the possibility of placental insufficiency.
- Epidural analgesia may be indicated because uterine contractions are often unusually painful.
- Continuous fetal heart rate monitoring is desirable.

Operative vaginal delivery

Assisted or operative (instrumental) vaginal delivery is used when the mother is unable to give birth without medical or surgical assistance. Assisted vaginal birth is a widely practised intervention, accounting for approximately 11% of births in the UK, and 15% in Australia and Canada. Women who use epidural analgesia are at increased risk of having an instrumental assisted birth.

Forceps method

Forceps are most commonly used to expedite the birth of the head or to protect the fetus or the mother, or both, from trauma and exhaustion. Forceps are also used to assist the delivery of the after-coming head of the breech.

Obstetric forceps are composed of two separate blades, right and left, that are inserted separately on each side of the head and then locked together. The blades are spoon shaped (cephalic curve) to accommodate the form of the baby's head.

Forceps deliveries fall into two categories, low- and mid-cavity and rotational. High-cavity forceps are now considered unsafe and a caesarean section will be carried out instead.

The main indications for a forceps delivery are delay in the second stage of labour, fetal compromise and maternal distress.

Prior to forceps delivery, ensure:

+ the woman's bladder is empty to prevent injury
+ adequate analgesia is provided (epidural, or pudendal block plus perineal infiltration of local anaesthetic)
+ information is given and consent obtained
+ paediatrician or advanced neonatal practitioner is informed and available if required
+ neonatal resuscitation equipment is checked and prepared in case it is necessary
+ fully dilated cervix
+ sufficient space in pelvis
+ membranes are ruptured

Ventouse method

The ventouse vacuum extractor is an instrument that applies traction. It can be used as an alternative to forceps. The cup clings to the fetal scalp by suction and is used to assist maternal effort. It may be used when there is a delay in labour, when the cervix is not quite fully dilated. It may also be useful in the case of a second twin, when the head remains relatively high.

Procedure

+ The woman is usually in the lithotomy position; the same precautions should be observed as for a forceps birth.
+ The cup of the ventouse is placed as near as possible to, or on, the flexing point of the fetal head.
+ The vacuum in the cup is gradually increased to achieve close application to the fetal head, usually to $0.8 \ kg/cm^2$.
+ When the vacuum is achieved, traction is applied with a contraction and with maternal effort. Traction is applied downwards and back-wards, then forwards and upwards, following the natural curve of the pelvis.
+ The vacuum is released and the cup is removed at the crowning of the fetal head.
+ The mother can then push the baby for the final part of the birth.

Complications

Prolonged traction will increase the likelihood of scalp abrasions, cephalohaematoma and subaponeurotic bleeding.

Further reading

Royal College of Obstetricians and Gynaecologists, 2011. Operative vaginal delivery. Green-top guideline no. 26. https://www.rcog. org.uk/en/guidelines-research-services/guidelines/gtg26/.

Ophthalmia neonatorum

Ophthalmia neonatorum is a notifiable condition. It involves a purulent discharge from the eyes of an infant that occurs within 21 days of birth. The condition is usually acquired during vaginal birth and causative organisms include

+ *Staphylococcus aureus*
+ *Streptococcus pneumoniae*
+ *Haemophilus influenzae*
+ *Escherichia coli*
+ *Klebsiella*
+ *Pseudomonas*
+ *Chlamydia trachomatis*
+ *Neisseria gonorrhoeae*

Chlamydia and gonorrhoea can cause conjunctival scarring, corneal infiltration, blindness and systemic spread.

Treatment involves local cleaning and care of the eyes with normal saline and appropriate drug therapy for the baby (and mother if required). See also Neonatal infections.

Opiate drugs   See Pain control.

Oxytocin

Oxytocin is a hormone produced by the hypothalamus. It plays a role in social bonding and sexual reproduction, as well as during and after childbirth. It can be used as a drug to cause contractions of the uterus to start or accelerate labour, and to decrease or stop bleeding after delivery. It also plays an essential role in stimulation of lactation, and bonding between mother and baby.

In induction of labour, oxytocin may be used in conjunction with artificial rupture of membranes (ARM). However, it may produce side effects such as hyperstimulation of the uterus, which could cause fetal hypoxia and uterine rupture, and water retention. Prolonged use may contribute to uterine atony postpartum.

Oxytocin can be used alone or in combination with ergometrine in the third stage of labour as a uterotonic, to assist delivery of the placenta and products of conception, and/or to control the risk of postpartum haemorrhage.

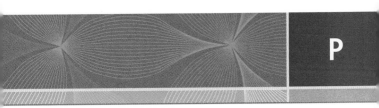

Pain

Pain is a complex interaction of physiological and psychological responses.

Nociceptive pain

Pain caused by actual or potential tissue damage (e.g., a cut, burn or other injury, arthritis) or pressure (e.g., from a tumour); activated or damaged nerve endings send pain messages to the brain. Tends to be sharp or aching.

Neuropathic pain

Pain caused by a problem with one or more nerves; pain messages are sent to the brain in the absence of injury or tissue damage. Often described as burning, stabbing or shooting; may be painful pins and needles, or electric-shock-like sensations; a light touch may be felt as painful (allodynia), mild discomfort may be felt as severe pain.

Pain in labour

The discomfort of labour is caused by the descent of the fetal head (or presenting part) further into the pelvis, by pressure on the cervix and the stretching of the vaginal walls and pelvic floor muscles as descent occurs. The large uterine muscle is contracting more strongly, more frequently and for a longer duration as labour progresses, increasing the discomfort felt by the woman.

The biological, psychological, social, spiritual, cultural and educational dimensions of each woman have an impact on how she expresses herself and how she perceives pain during labour. Emotions such as fear and anxiety affect her perception of pain.

Midwives should work with women to encourage them to maintain control and be as mobile as possible throughout labour. Mobility in labour lessens the need for analgesia. Pain control during labour should be woman-centred, not medically oriented. (For pharmacological and nonpharmacological methods of pain control, see Pain control.)

Pain control

A clear distinction should be made between the traditional goal of pain relief and control of pain in labour. The aim should be to give the woman control of pain rather than trying to eradicate it. This may require a multifaceted approach that includes pharmacological and nonpharmacological methods.

Nonpharmacological methods of pain control

- Breathing and relaxation techniques
- Massage
- Hydrotherapy
- Aromatherapy
- Transcutaneous electrical nerve stimulation (TENS)
- Reflexology
- Homeopathy
- Music therapy
- Acupuncture
- Herbal medicine

A Cochrane review of studies involving acupuncture, acupressure, aromatherapy, massage and relaxation techniques found that acupuncture reduced the need for analgesia; women taught self-hypnosis had decreased need for pharmacological analgesia; and no differences were seen for women receiving aromatherapy. Few other complementary therapies have been subjected to scientific study. In the UK, the National Institute for Health and Care Excellence (NICE) suggests that breathing and relaxation techniques, and massage, may be helpful and have no side effects. Women should be offered the option of being in water during labour as this helps with pain. Acupuncture, acupressure or hypnosis are not available on the National Health Service (NHS), but women can use these techniques if they wish. Starting to use a TENS machine once the woman is in established labour will not help with pain.

Pharmacological methods of pain control

- Opiate drugs: frequently used during childbirth because of their powerful analgesic properties. The most commonly used are those listed below. All have similar pain-relieving properties, but they also have side effects, including nausea, vomiting and drowsiness in the mother, and depression of the baby's respiratory centre at birth.
  - Pethidine: usually administered intramuscularly in doses of 50–150 mg; takes about 20 minutes to have an effect
  - Diamorphine: usual dose is 10 mg given via intramuscular injection
  - Meptazinol: usually given in doses of 100–150 mg intramuscularly
- Inhalation analgesia: the most commonly used inhalation analgesia in labour is a premixed gas comprising up to 50% nitrous oxide and 50% oxygen, administered through a piped system or via an Entonox apparatus. It takes effect within 20 seconds, with maximum efficacy occurring after about 45–50 seconds.
- Regional (epidural) analgesia: A local anaesthetic is injected into the epidural space of the lumbar region, usually between vertebrae L1 and L2, or L2 and L3, or between L3 and L4. Continuous infusion of local anaesthetic (bupivacaine) and opioids (usually fentanyl) is administered via a syringe pump. Midwives top up the epidural block by giving a further dose as prescribed by the anaesthetist. The midwife is personally responsible for ensuring she is competent to carry out the procedure, and should be aware of possible complications and their immediate treatment.

Further reading

NICE, 2014. Intrapartum care for healthy women and babies. Clinical guideline CG190. https://www.nice.org.uk/guidance/cg190.

Royal College of Midwives, 2012. Evidence based guidelines for midwifery-led care in labour: understanding pharmacological pain relief. https://www.rcm.org.uk/sites/default/files/Understanding%20Pharmacological%20Pain%20Relief_0.pdf.

Tidy, C., 2015. Pain relief in labour. Professional reference. http://patient.info/doctor/pain-relief-in-labour.

Pelvic floor

The pelvic floor is formed by the soft tissues that fill the outlet of the pelvis. The most important of these is the diaphragm of muscle slung like a hammock from the walls of the pelvis, through which pass the urethra, vagina and anal canal. Exercising pelvic floor muscles antenatally can help them to retain their function (supporting the bladder, uterus and bowel) and can help the muscles relax during parturition. Women should be encouraged to resume pelvic floor exercises as soon as they can after the birth in order to regain bladder control, prevent incontinence and prolapse, and to ensure normal sexual satisfaction for both partners in the future.

Perinatal mental health

Stress/anxiety and domestic abuse

Women are affected emotionally and socially on many levels. Women in abusive relationships are particularly vulnerable. Approximately 30% of domestic violence and abuse begins or escalates during pregnancy or following childbirth.

The transition to motherhood

Postnatally, parents may find coping with the demands of a new baby, infant feeding, financial constraints and adjusting to changes in roles and relationships particularly testing emotionally. Disturbed sleep is inevitable. Soreness and pain from perineal trauma will affect libido; so too will the feelings of exhaustion, despair and unhappiness that may be associated with the round-the-clock demands of caring for a new baby.

Normal emotional changes during pregnancy, labour and the puerperium

It is perfectly normal for women to have periods of self-doubt and crises of confidence. They may experience fluctuations between positive and negative emotions, as described below.

First trimester

+ Pleasure, excitement, elation
+ Dismay, disappointment
+ Ambivalence
+ Emotional lability
+ Increased femininity

Second trimester

+ A feeling of wellbeing
+ A sense of increased attachment to the fetus
+ Stress and anxiety about antenatal screening and diagnostic tests
+ Increased demand for knowledge and information

+ Feelings relating to the need for increasing detachment from work commitments

Third trimester

+ Loss of or increased libido
+ Altered body image
+ Psychological effects from physiological discomforts such as backache and heartburn
+ Anxiety about labour (e.g., pain)
+ Anxiety about fetal abnormality
+ Increased vulnerability to major life events

Labour

For many women, labour will be greeted with varied emotional responses such as:

+ great excitement and anticipation to utter dread
+ fear of the unknown
+ fear of technology, intervention
+ fear of hospitals, illness and death
+ tension, fear and anxiety about pain and lack of control
+ concerns about the baby and ability of their partner to support/cope
+ a fear of lack of privacy or embarrassment

Women's perceptions of control during labour are influenced by:

+ continuity of care by the midwife
+ one-to-one care in labour
+ not being left for long periods
+ being involved in decision making

The puerperium

Normal emotional changes are complex and may encompass the following:

+ relief labour is over—others may convey a cool detachment from events
+ contradictory and conflicting feelings from joy and elation to exhaustion and helplessness
+ closeness to partner and/or baby or lack of interest
+ desire for prolonged skin-to-skin contact and early breastfeeding
+ fear of the unknown and realization of overwhelming responsibility
+ exhaustion and increased emotionality
+ pain (e.g., perineal, nipples)
+ increased vulnerability and indecisiveness
+ loss of libido, disturbed sleep, anxiety

Postnatal 'blues'

This normal and transient phase is experienced by 50%–80%, of women depending on parity. The onset typically occurs between 3 and 4 days postpartum, but may last up to a week or more, though rarely persisting for longer than a few days. The features of this state are mild and transitory and may include a state in which women usually experience labile emotions. The actual aetiology is unclear but hormonal influences seem to be implicated, as the period of increased emotionality appears to coincide with the production of milk. Although the condition is self limiting, the midwife must be vigilant as persistent features could be indicative of depressive illness.

Emotional distress associated with traumatic birth events

Over recent years the label 'posttraumatic stress disorder' (PTSD) has emerged in midwifery practice. Many women will eventually overcome the stress, pain and trauma that might have been their birth experience. However, others may find their birth experience blights their life and affects relationships with their partner and baby.

Perinatal psychiatric disorders

Perinatal psychiatric disorders encompass those that develop during the perinatal period as well as preexisting disorders. Midwives are recommended to routinely ask at early pregnancy assessment about previous mental health problems, their severity and care. For example:

+ During the past months, have you often been bothered by feeling down, depressed or hopeless?
+ During the past months, have you often been bothered by having little interest or pleasure in doing things?

A third question should be considered if the woman answers 'yes' to initial question:

+ Is this something you feel you need or want help with?

Types of psychiatric disorder

Psychiatric disorders are conventionally grouped into the following categories:

+ serious mental illness, e.g., schizophrenia, bipolar illness, depressive illness
+ mild to moderate psychiatric disorders, e.g., mild to moderate depressive illness, anxiety disorders, panic disorders, obsessive compulsive disorder, PTSD
+ adjustment reactions, e.g., distressing reactions to death, adversity

- substance misuse, e.g., dependence on alcohol or drugs
- personality disorders—should only be used for those with persistent severe problems, e.g., maintaining satisfactory relationships, controlling their behaviour
- learning disability—when people have lifetime evidence of intellectual and cognitive impairment

Psychiatric disorder in pregnancy

New onset of psychiatric disorder in pregnancy is mostly accounted for by mild depressive illness, mixed anxiety and depression or anxiety states. Most conditions are likely to improve as pregnancy progresses. Caution needs to be exercised before pharmacological intervention.

New onset psychosis in pregnancy is relatively rare but if the condition appears it requires urgent and expert treatment.

Preexisting psychiatric disorders require individualized care plans.

- Well, stable, not on medication—risk of becoming psychotic postnatally
- Relatively well and stable but taking medication—need expert advice on risks and benefits of treatment
- Chronically mentally ill and on medication—need careful monitoring by maternity, psychiatric and social services

Psychiatric disorders after birth

Conventionally, three postpartum disorders are described:

- the 'blues'
- puerperal psychosis
- postnatal depression

The 'blues'

The blues is a common dysphoric, self-limiting state, occurring in the first week postpartum.

Puerperal psychosis

This is the most severe form of postpartum affective disorder. The onset is very sudden, the majority presenting in the first 14 days postpartum, most commonly between day 3 and day 7.

Features may include:

- restlessness and agitation
- confusion and perplexity
- suspicion and fear, even terror
- insomnia
- episodes of mania making the woman hyperactive (e.g., talking rapidly and incessantly, and being very overactive and elated)

- neglect of basic needs (e.g., nutrition and hydration)
- hallucinations and morbid delusional thoughts involving self and baby
- major behavioural disturbance
- profound depressive mood

Care and management should be based on:

- preventive measures preconception/antenatally
- interprofessional collaboration
- care in a specialist mother and baby unit

Postnatal depressive illness

The term postnatal depression should only be used for a nonpsychotic depressive illness of mild to moderate severity, which arises within 3 months of childbirth.

Where a screening tool such as the Edinburgh Postnatal Depression Scale is used, a score of 14 is said to correlate with a clinical diagnosis of major depression.

Severe postnatal depression is an early-onset condition that develops over 2–4 weeks, unlike the abrupt onset of puerperal psychosis. The more severe illnesses tend to present by 4–6 weeks postpartum but the majority tend to present later, between 8 and 12 weeks postpartum.

The main characteristics are the following:

- 'biological syndrome' of sleep disturbance—waking early in the morning—the woman will feel most depressed and her symptoms will be worst at the start of the day
- impaired concentration, disturbed thought processes, indecisiveness and an inability to cope with everyday life
- emotional detachment and profound lowering of mood
- loss of ability to feel pleasure (anhedonia)
- feelings of guilt, incompetence and of being a 'bad' mother
- in approximately one-third of women, distressing intrusive obsessional thoughts and ruminations
- commonly, extreme anxiety and even panic attacks
- impaired appetite and weight loss
- in a small number, a depressive psychosis and morbid, delusional thoughts and hallucinations

Treatment of perinatal psychiatric disorders

There are three components to management:

- psychological treatment and social intervention
- pharmacological treatment
- services and resources

Some or all will be required.

Pharmacological treatment

Given that there is a paucity of systematic research into the efficacy and risks of pharmacological intervention in the management of perinatal mental illness, balancing risk to the fetus/baby against the risk of not treating the mother is a challenge. Women should be actively supported to breastfeed their baby, if this is their wish.

General principles

- Whenever possible, conception and birth should be medication free.
- Most new episodes of mental illness in pregnancy occur early and improve as pregnancy progresses with appropriate psychosocial interventions.
- Liaison between the midwife, GP, obstetrician, psychiatrist, community psychiatric nurse, health visitor and, where necessary, social worker is of great importance.
- No medication is of proven safety.
- Medications that carry a significant risk of teratogenesis have been shown to affect 1–2% of exposed pregnancies, so may be considered of low risk. Nevertheless they may contribute to fetal demise, intrauterine growth restriction, organ dysgenesis and adverse effects on the neonate, such as withdrawal.
- Serious mental illness requires robust treatment; the more serious the illness is, the more likely it is that the risks of not treating outweigh the risks of treating.
- Babies more than 12 weeks old are at low risk of exposure to antidepressants in breast milk.
- Breast milk levels will reflect the serum levels of the medication. Therefore women should be advised to avoid feeding at times of peak plasma level, and preferably should time their medication after a feed and before the baby's longest sleep.
- The baby should be monitored for any deleterious effects, particularly weight gain and drowsiness.

Further reading/resources

Maternal Mental Health: Everyone's business. http://everyonesbusiness.org.uk/?page_id=6.

Maternal Mental Health Alliance. http://maternalmentalhealthalliance.org.

Continued

Further reading/resources—cont'd

National Institute for Health and Care Excellence, 2014, updated June
2015. Antenatal and postnatal mental health: clinical
management and service guidance. Clinical guideline 192. https://
www.nice.org.uk/guidance/cg192.

Royal College of General Practitioners. Perinatal mental health toolkit.
http://www.rcgp.org.uk/clinical-and-research/toolkits/perinatal-
mental-health-toolkit.aspx.

World Health Organization. Maternal mental health. http://www.
who.int/mental_health/maternal-child/maternal_mental_health/
en/.

Perineum

The perineum is the region between the vulva and the anus. In the second
stage of labour, the perineum distends as the baby's head descends towards
the vulva. The majority of women who have a vaginal birth will sustain
some degree of perineal trauma, either from a spontaneous perineal tear
or episiotomy or both. (See Episiotomy.)

Perineal trauma

Spontaneous trauma may be of the labia anteriorly, the perineum posteriorly
or both. A gentle, thorough examination must be carried out to assess the
extent of the trauma accurately and to determine who should carry out
the repair.

+ *Anterior labial tears.* A suture may be necessary to secure haemostasis.
+ *Posterior perineal trauma.* Usually classified in degrees. Third- and
  fourth-degree tears should be repaired by an experienced obstetrician,
  under general anaesthetic or effective epidural or spinal anaesthesia.
  + A first-degree tear involves the fourchette only.
  + A second-degree tear involves the fourchette and the perineal muscles.
  + A third-degree tear involves the fourchette, the perineal muscles
    and the anal sphincter.
  + A fourth-degree tear is sometimes used to describe trauma that
    extends into the rectal mucosa.

Further reading

Royal College of Midwives, 2012. Evidence based guidelines for
midwifery-led care in labour: care of the perineum. https://www.
rcm.org.uk/sites/default/files/Care%20of%20the%20Perineum.
pdf.

Phototherapy

Phototherapy is used in the management of jaundice to prevent the concentration of unconjugated bilirubin in the blood from reaching levels where neurotoxicity may occur. The neonate's skin is exposed to high-intensity light, which photochemically converts fat-soluble unconjugated bilirubin into water-soluble bilirubin that can be excreted in bile and urine. Treatment may be intermittent or continuous and interrupted only for essential care.

Side effects of treatment include hyperthermia, dehydration, damage to the retina, rashes and skin burns, decreased calcium levels, low platelet counts and increased red cell osmotic fragility. In addition, the baby may experience alterations in infant state and neurobehavioural organization, as well as isolation and lack of usual sensory experiences including visual deprivation.

Further reading

Kelly, M.A., 2014. Neonatal jaundice and phototherapy. Great Ormond Street Hospital for Children guideline. http://www.gosh.nhs.uk/health-professionals/clinical-guidelines/jaundice-management-neonates.

National Institute for Health and Care Excellence, 2010, updated May 2016. Jaundice in newborn babies under 28 days. Clinical guideline 98. https://www.nice.org.uk/guidance/cg98.

Placenta

The placenta (Fig. 25) is the flattened circular organ in the uterus of pregnant women (and indeed other mammals) which links closely to the mother's circulation to carry out functions that the fetus is unable to perform for itself during intrauterine life. It provides oxygen and nutrients to the fetus, and removes waste products such as carbon dioxide, returning them to the maternal circulation for elimination. The placenta also produces hormones that aid the growth and development of the fetus, and provides some protection against bacterial infection.

At term the placenta is about 20 cm in diameter and 2.5 cm thick. The maternal surface is arranged in about 20 cotyledons (lobes) made up of lobules, each of which contains a single villus with its branches. The fetal surface is covered in amnion, which gives it a white, shiny appearance. Branches of the umbilical vein and arteries are visible, spreading out from the insertion of the umbilical cord.

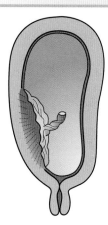

Fig. 25 The placenta.

Delivery of the placenta

During the third stage of labour, separation and expulsion of the placenta and membranes occurs. The placenta may shear off during the final expulsive contractions accompanying the birth of the baby, or remain adherent for some considerable time. The third stage usually lasts between 5 and 15 minutes, but any period up to 1 hour may be considered within normal limits.

On delivery of the placenta and membranes (products of conception), they should be examined as soon as possible so that, if there is any doubt about their completeness, further action can be taken. Retained products of conception are one of the main causes of postpartum haemorrhage and infection.

Retained placenta

A diagnosis is reached when the placenta remains undelivered after a specified period of time (up to 1 hour following the baby's birth). Conventional treatment is to separate the placenta from the uterine wall digitally, effecting a manual removal.

- Placenta accreta: abnormally adherent placenta into the muscle layer of the uterus
- Placenta increta: abnormally adherent placenta into the perimetrium of the uterus
- Placenta percreta: abnormally adherent placenta through the muscle layer of the uterus

- Placenta praevia: a condition in which some or all of the placenta is attached in the lower segment of the uterus
- Placental abruption (abruptio placentae): premature separation of a normally situated placenta. The term is normally used from viability (24 weeks). Any woman with a history suggestive of placental abruption needs urgent medical attention.

Further reading

National Institute for Health and Care Excellence, 2014. Intrapartum care for healthy women and babies. Clinical guideline 190. https://www.nice.org.uk/guidance/cg190/chapter/1-recommendations.

Royal College of Midwives, 2012. Evidence based guidelines for midwifery-led care in labour: third stage of labour. https://www.rcm.org.uk/sites/default/files/Third%20Stage%20of%20Labour.pdf.

Royal College of Obstetricians and Gynaecologists, 2011. Placenta praevia, placenta praevia accreta and vasa praevia: diagnosis and management. Green-top guideline no. 27. https://www.rcog.org.uk/globalassets/documents/guidelines/gtg_27.pdf.

Placenta praevia

A condition in which the placenta is partially or wholly implanted in the lower uterine segment on either the anterior or posterior wall.

Type 1 (Fig. 26)

- The majority of the placenta is in the upper uterine segment
- Blood loss is usually mild and the mother and fetus remain in good condition
- Vaginal birth is possible

Type 2 (Fig. 27)

- The placenta is partially located in the lower segment near the internal cervical os
- Blood loss is usually moderate, although the conditions of the mother and fetus can vary
- Vaginal birth is possible, particularly if the placenta is anterior

Type 3 (Fig. 28)

- The placenta is located over the internal cervical os but not centrally
- Bleeding is likely to be severe
- Vaginal birth is inappropriate

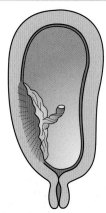

Fig. 26 Placenta preavia (type 1).

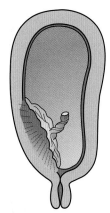

Fig. 27 Placenta praevia (type 2).

Type 4 (Fig. 29)
+ The placenta is located centrally over the internal cervical os
+ Torrential haemorrhage is very likely
+ Caesarean section is essential

Postnatal care

Defining the puerperium and the postnatal period

Following the birth of the baby and expulsion of the placenta, the mother enters a period of physical and psychological recuperation. From a medical

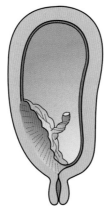

Fig. 28 **Placenta praevia (type 3).**

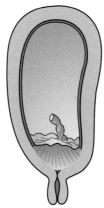

Fig. 29 **Placenta praevia (type 4).**

and physiological viewpoint this period, called the *puerperium*, starts immediately after delivery of the placenta and membranes and continues for 6 weeks.

Midwives and the management of postpartum care

The *postnatal period* means the period after the end of labour during which the attendance of a midwife upon the woman and baby is required, being not less than 10 days and for a longer period if the midwife considers it necessary (Nursing and Midwifery Council [NMC] Rule).

Immediate care

It is advisable for mother and infant to remain in the midwife's care for at least an hour after birth, regardless of the birth setting.

+ The woman should be encouraged to pass urine because a full bladder may impede uterine contraction.
+ Uterine contraction and blood loss should be checked on several occasions in the first hour.
+ Throughout this same period the midwife should pay regard to the baby's general wellbeing. She should check the security of the cord clamp and observe general skin colour, respirations and temperature.
+ The warmest place for a baby is to be placed in a direct skin-to-skin contact position with the mother, or wrapped and cuddled, whichever she prefers.
+ Most women intending to breastfeed will wish to put their baby to the breast during the first moments of contact.

Once the placenta is expelled, a number of physiological processes take place and the uterus returns to its non-pregnant state (involution). The midwife should undertake immediate and then regular observations of fundal height and the degree of uterine contraction in the first few hours after birth. On abdominal palpation, the fundus of the uterus should be located centrally, at the same level or slightly below the umbilicus, and should feel firm. A well-contracted uterus will gradually reduce in size until it is no longer palpable above the symphysis pubis. It should not feel tender, although the woman may experience afterpains.

The observations obtained by the midwife about the state of involution of the uterus should be placed into context alongside the colour, amount and duration of the woman's vaginal fluid loss and her general state of health at that time.

Postpartum vaginal fluid loss (lochia)

Blood products constitute the major part of the vaginal loss immediately after the birth of the baby and expulsion of the placenta. As involution progresses, the vaginal loss reflects this and changes from a predominantly fresh blood loss to one that contains stale blood products, lanugo, vernix and other debris from the unwanted products of the conception. This loss varies from woman to woman, being lighter or darker in colour, but for any woman the shade and density tend to be consistent.

Assessment of vaginal blood loss

The mother should be asked about the current vaginal loss:

+ whether this is more or less than previously
+ whether it is lighter or darker than previously
+ whether she herself has any concerns about it

It is of particular importance to record any clots passed and when these occurred.

Perineal pain

Regardless of whether the birth resulted in actual perineal trauma, women are likely to feel bruised around the vaginal and perineal tissues for the first few days after the birth. Women who have undergone any degree of actual perineal injury will experience pain for several days until healing takes place.

All women should be asked about discomfort in the perineal area, regardless of whether there is a record of actual perineal trauma. Where women appear to have no discomfort or anxieties about their perineum, it is not essential for the midwife to examine this area. For the majority of women, the perineal wound gradually becomes less painful and healing should occur by 7–10 days after the birth.

Appropriate information and advice are important components in pain management and should take into account women's individual experiences of their pain and their preferences for its relief.

Women may find soaking in a bath of great comfort to them regardless of any additive, and relief may be derived from the use of a bidet or cool water poured over the area that is tender.

Vital signs and general health

Observations of pulse, temperature, respiration and blood pressure

While monitoring the pulse rate the midwife can also observe a number of related signs of wellbeing, as well as just listening to what the woman is saying:

+ respiratory rate
+ overall body temperature
+ any untoward body odour
+ skin condition
+ overall colour and complexion

Observation of temperature is unnecessary in women who are well and without symptoms that could be associated with an infection. Where the woman complains of feeling unwell with flulike symptoms, or there are signs of possible infection, then the temperature must be taken.

Blood pressure

Following the birth of the baby, a baseline recording of the woman's blood pressure will be made. In the absence of any previous history of morbidity associated with hypertension, it is usual for the blood pressure to return to a normal range within 24 hours of the birth. Routine observations of blood pressure is not required.

Circulation

The body has to reabsorb a quantity of excess fluid following the birth. For the majority of women this results in passing large quantities of urine, particularly in the first day, as diuresis is increased. Women may also experience oedema of their ankles and feet and this swelling may be greater than that experienced in pregnancy. These are variations of normal physiological processes and should resolve within the puerperal time scale as the woman's activity levels also increase. Advice should be related to:

+ taking reasonable exercise
+ avoiding long periods of standing
+ elevating the feet and legs when sitting, where possible

Swollen ankles should be bilateral and not accompanied by pain; the midwife should note particularly if this is present in one calf only, as it could indicate a deep vein thrombosis.

Skin and nutrition

Women who have suffered from urticaria of pregnancy or cholestasis of the liver should experience relief once the pregnancy is over. The pace of life once the baby is born might lead to women having a reduced fluid intake than formerly or to taking a different diet. This in turn might affect their skin and overall physiological state. Women should be encouraged to maintain a balanced fluid intake and to eat a diet that has a greater proportion of fresh food in it.

Urine and bowel function

Minor disorders of urinary and bowel function are common. These may be associated with retention or incontinence of urine or constipation, or both. The midwife should explore the possible cause of this and decide whether it will resolve spontaneously or requires further investigation.

Exercise and healthy activity versus rest, relaxation and sleep

Exploring each woman's level of activity will encourage advice in relation to appropriate exercise and, by association, nutritional intake and rest or relaxation and sleep. Undertaking regular pelvic floor exercises is of benefit to women's long-term health.

Afterpains

Management of afterpains is by an appropriate analgesic; where possible, this should be taken prior to breastfeeding, as it is the production of oxytocin in relation to the let-down response that initiates the contraction in the uterus and causes pain. Pain in the uterus that is constant or present on abdominal palpation is unlikely to be associated with afterpains and further enquiry should be made. Women might also confuse afterpains with flatus pain, especially after an operative birth or where they are constipated. Relief of the cause is likely to relieve the symptoms.

Future health, future fertility

Midwives need to be aware of a range of different needs with regard to women's sexuality and should be able to offer sensitive and appropriate advice on contraception where this is needed.

Further reading

National Institute for Health and Care Excellence, 2006, updated 2015. Postnatal care up to 8 weeks after birth. Clinical guideline 37. https://www.nice.org.uk/guidance/cg37.
Royal College of Midwives, 2014. Postnatal care planning. https://www.rcm.org.uk/sites/default/files/Pressure%20Points%20-%20Postnatal%20Care%20Planning%20-%20Web%20Copy.pdf.

Postnatal depression

Postnatal depression is a nonpsychotic depressive illness of mild to moderate severity arising within 3 months of childbirth.

Main characteristics are:

* diurnal mood changes and sleep disturbance—waking early in the morning; the woman will feel most depressed and her symptoms will be worse at the start of the day;
* impaired concentration, disturbed thought processes, indecisiveness and an inability to cope with everyday life;
* emotional detachment and profound lowering of mood;
* loss of ability to feel pleasure (anhedonia);
* feelings of guilt, incompetence and of being a 'bad' mother;
* in approximately one-third of women, distressing, intrusive obsessional thoughts;

+ commonly, extreme anxiety and even panic attacks;
+ impaired appetite and weight loss;
+ in a small number, depressive psychosis, morbid, delusional thoughts and hallucinations.

The Edinburgh Postnatal Depression Scale is a useful screening tool but can lead to 'false positives' and medicalization of low mood and situational distress, and should not replace clinical judgement.

Further reading

Association for Postnatal Illness. Postnatal depression. http://apni. org/leaflets/post-natal-depression/.

Edinburgh Postnatal Depression Scale: https://psychology-tools.com/ epds/.

MIND. Postnatal depression and perinatal mental health. http://www. mind.org.uk/information-support/types-of-mental-health-problems/postnatal-depression-and-perinatal-mental-health/ #.V9wCfmPcHiR.

Royal College of Midwives, 2014. Maternal mental health. Improving emotional wellbeing in postnatal care. https://www.rcm.org.uk/ sites/default/files/Pressure%20Points%20-%20Mental%20 Health%20-%20Final_0.pdf.

Postpartum haemorrhage

Postpartum haemorrhage (PPH) is defined as excessive bleeding from the genital tract at any time following the baby's birth up to 12 weeks after birth.

+ If it occurs during the third stage of labour or within 24 hours of delivery, it is termed *primary postpartum haemorrhage*.
+ If it occurs subsequent to the first 24 hours following birth up until the 12th week postpartum, it is termed *secondary postpartum haemorrhage*.

Primary postpartum haemorrhage

A measured loss that reaches 500 mL or any loss that adversely affects the mother's condition constitutes a PPH.

There are several reasons why a PPH may occur, including:

+ atonic uterus
+ retained placenta
+ trauma
+ blood coagulation disorder

Atonic uterus

This is a failure of the myometrium at the placental site to contract and retract, and to compress torn blood vessels and control blood loss by a living ligature action. Causes of atonic uterine action resulting in PPH are:

- incomplete separation of the placenta
- retained cotyledon, placental fragment or membranes
- precipitate labour
- prolonged labour resulting in uterine inertia
- polyhydramnios or multiple pregnancy causing overdistension of uterine muscle
- placenta praevia
- placental abruption
- general anaesthesia, especially halothane or cyclopropane
- mismanagement of the third stage of labour
- a full bladder
- aetiology unknown

There are, in addition, a number of factors that do not directly *cause* a PPH, but do increase the likelihood of excessive bleeding:

- previous history of PPH or retained placenta
- high parity, resulting in uterine scar tissue
- presence of fibroids
- maternal anaemia
- ketoacidosis
- multiple pregnancy

Signs of primary postpartum haemorrhage

These may be obvious, such as visible bleeding or maternal collapse, or more subtle, such as pallor, rising pulse rate, falling blood pressure, altered level of consciousness. The mother may become restless or drowsy, and have an enlarged uterus that feels 'boggy' on palpation (i.e., soft, distended and lacking tone), even if little blood loss is visible.

Prophylaxis

- During the antenatal period, identify risk factors, e.g., previous obstetric history, anaemia
- During labour, prevent prolonged labour and ketoacidosis
- Ensure the mother does not have a full bladder at any stage
- Give prophylactic administration of a uterotonic agent
- If a woman is known to have a placenta praevia keep 2 units of cross-matched blood available

Management of primary postpartum haemorrhage (Fig. 30)

There are three basic principles of care.

+ Call for medical aid
+ Stop the bleeding
  + Rub up a contraction
  + Give a uterotonic
  + Empty the bladder
  + Empty the uterus
  + Apply pressure if there is trauma
+ Resuscitate the mother

Secondary or delayed primary postpartum haemorrhage

This is where there is excessive or prolonged vaginal loss from 24 hours after delivery of the placenta and for up to 12 weeks postpartum. Unlike primary PPH, which includes a specified volume of blood loss as part of its definition, there is no such volume defined for secondary PPH.

Regardless of the timing of any haemorrhage, it is most frequently the placental site that is the source. Alternatively, a cervical or deep vaginal wall tear or trauma to the perineum might be the cause in women who have recently given birth. Retained placental fragments or other products of conception are likely to inhibit the process of involution, or reopen the placental wound. The diagnosis is likely to be determined by the woman's condition and pattern of events and is also often complicated by the presence of infection.

Signs of secondary PPH

+ Lochial loss is heavier than normal
+ Lochia returns to a bright red loss and may be offensive
+ Subinvolution of the uterus
+ Pyrexia and tachycardia
+ Haematoma formation

Treatment

+ Call a doctor
+ Reassure the woman and her support person(s)
+ Rub up a contraction by massaging the uterus if it is still palpable
+ Express any clots
+ Encourage the mother to empty her bladder
+ Give a uterotonic drug, such as ergometrine maleate, by the intravenous or intramuscular route
+ Keep all pads and linen to assess the volume of blood lost

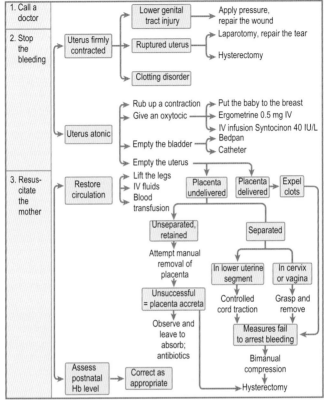

Fig. 30 Management of primary postpartum haemorrhage.

+ Antibiotics may be prescribed
+ If retained products of conception are seen on an ultrasound scan, it may be appropriate to transfer the woman to hospital and prepare her for theatre

Preeclampsia

Preeclampsia is a condition peculiar to pregnancy, which is characterized by hypertension, proteinuria and systemic dysfunction.

Preeclampsia is diagnosed on the basis of hypertension with proteinuria, when proteinuria is measured as >1+ on dipstick or >0.3 g/L of protein in a random clean catch specimen or an excretion of 0.3 g of protein/24 hours.

In the absence of proteinuria, preeclampsia is suspected when hypertension is accompanied by symptoms including:

+ headache
+ blurred vision
+ abdominal/epigastric pain, or
+ altered biochemistry: specifically, low platelet counts, abnormal liver enzyme levels

These signs and symptoms, together with blood pressure above 160 mmHg systolic or above 110 mmHg diastolic and proteinuria of 2+ or 3+ on a dipstick, demonstrate the more severe form of the disease.

Early detection and appropriate management can minimize the severity of the condition. A comprehensive history will identify:

+ adverse social circumstances or poverty, which could prevent the woman from attending for regular antenatal care
+ the mother's age and parity
+ primipaternity and partner-related factors
+ a family history of hypertensive disorders
+ a past history of preeclampsia
+ the presence of underlying medical disorders: for example, renal disease, diabetes, systemic lupus erythematosus (SLE) and thromboembolic disorders.

The two essential features of preeclampsia, hypertension and proteinuria, are assessed for at regular intervals throughout pregnancy. Diagnosis is usually based on the rise in blood pressure and the presence of proteinuria after 20 weeks' gestation.

Blood pressure measurement

The mother's blood pressure is taken early in pregnancy to compare with all subsequent recordings, taking into account the normal pattern in pregnancy. It is important to consider several factors in assessing blood pressure. Blood pressure machines should be calibrated for use in pregnancy and regularly maintained.

Blood pressure can be overestimated as a result of using a sphygmomanometer cuff of inadequate size relative to the arm circumference. The length of the bladder should be at least 80% of the arm circumference. Two cuffs should be available with inflation bladders of 35 cm for normal use and 42 cm for large arms.

Rounding off of blood pressure measurements should be avoided and an attempt should be made to record the blood pressure as accurately as possible to the nearest 2 mmHg.

The use of Korotkoff V (disappearance of sound) as a measure of the diastolic blood pressure has been found to be easier to obtain, more reproducible and closer to the intraarterial pressure; therefore, this reading should be used unless the sound is near zero, in which case Korotkoff IV (muffling sound) should be used instead.

Urinalysis

Proteinuria in the absence of urinary tract infection is indicative of glomerular endotheliosis. The amount of protein in the urine is frequently taken as an index of the severity of preeclampsia. A significant increase in proteinuria, coupled with diminished urinary output, indicates renal impairment. A 24-hour urine collection for total protein measurement will be required to be certain about the presence or absence of proteinuria and to provide an accurate quantitative assessment of protein loss. A finding of >300 mg/24 hours is considered to be indicative of mild to moderate preeclampsia and >3 g/24 hours is considered to be severe.

Oedema

The sudden severe widespread appearance of oedema is suggestive of preeclampsia or some underlying pathology and further investigations are necessary. This oedema pits on pressure and may be found in nondependent anatomical areas such as the face, hands, lower abdomen, and vulval and sacral areas.

Laboratory tests

Alterations in the following haematological and biochemical parameters are suggestive of preeclampsia:

+ increased haemoglobin (Hb) and haematocrit levels
+ thrombocytopenia
+ prolonged clotting times
+ raised serum creatinine and urea levels
+ raised serum uric acid level
+ abnormal liver function tests, particularly raised transaminases

Care and management

The aim of care is to monitor the condition of the woman and her fetus and, if possible, to prevent the hypertensive disorder worsening by using appropriate interventions and treatment. The objective is to prolong the pregnancy until the fetus is sufficiently mature to survive, while safeguarding the mother's life.

Antenatal care

Rest

It is preferable for the woman to rest at home and to be visited regularly by the midwife or GP. When proteinuria develops in addition to hypertension, the risks to the mother and fetus are considerably increased. Admission to hospital is required to monitor and evaluate the maternal and fetal condition.

Diet

There is little evidence to support dietary intervention for preventing or restricting the advance of preeclampsia.

Weight gain

Weight gain may be useful for monitoring the progression of preeclampsia in conjunction with other parameters.

Blood pressure and urinalysis

The blood pressure is monitored daily at home or every 4 hours when in hospital. Urine should be tested for protein daily. If protein is found in a midstream specimen of urine, a 24-hour urine collection is instigated in order to determine the amount of protein. The level of protein indicates the degree of vascular damage. Reduced kidney perfusion is indicated by:

* proteinuria
* reduced creatinine clearance
* increased serum creatinine and uric acid

Abdominal examination

This is carried out daily. Any discomfort or tenderness may be a sign of placental abruption. Upper abdominal pain is highly significant and indicative of haemolysis, elevated liver enzyme levels and low platelet levels (HELLP syndrome) associated with fulminating (rapid-onset) preeclampsia.
See HELLP syndrome.

Fetal assessment

It is advisable to undertake a biophysical profile in order to determine fetal health and wellbeing. This is done by the use of:

* kick charts
* cardiotocography (CTG) monitoring
* serial ultrasound scans to check for fetal growth
* assessment of liquor volume and fetal breathing movements or Doppler flow studies, or both, to determine placental blood flow.

Laboratory studies

These include:

- full blood count, platelet count and clotting profile
- urea and electrolytes
- creatinine and liver function tests, including albumin levels

In severe preeclampsia blood samples should be taken every 12–24 hours.

Antihypertensive therapy

The use of antihypertensive therapy as prophylaxis is controversial, as this shows no benefit in significantly prolonging pregnancy or improving maternal or fetal outcome. Its use is, however, advocated as short-term therapy in order to prevent an increase in blood pressure and the development of severe hypertension, thereby reducing the risk to the mother of cerebral haemorrhage. Methyldopa is the most widely used drug in women with mild to moderate gestational hypertension and appears to be safe and effective for both mother and fetus.

Alpha and beta blockers such as labetalol are considered safe in pregnancy. Atenolol used over the long term is not recommended as it may cause significant fetal growth restriction.

Antithrombotic agents

Early activation of the clotting system may contribute to the later pathology of preeclampsia; as a result, the use of anticoagulants or antiplatelet agents has been considered for the prevention of preeclampsia and fetal growth restriction. Aspirin is thought to inhibit the production of the platelet-aggregating agent, thromboxane A_2; it is recommended for women at risk from 12 weeks.

Intrapartum care

It is essential to monitor the maternal and fetal condition carefully.

Vital signs

Blood pressure is measured half-hourly, or every 15–20 minutes in severe preeclampsia.

Because of the potentially rapid haemodynamic changes in preeclampsia, a number of authors recommend the measurement of the mean arterial pressure (MAP). MAP reflects the systemic perfusion pressure, and therefore the degree of hypovolaemia, whereas manual measurement of diastolic pressure alone is a better indicator of the degree of hypertension.

Observation of the respiratory rate (>14/min) will be complemented with pulse oximetry in severe preeclampsia; this gives an indication of the degree of maternal hypoxia.

Temperature should be recorded as necessary.

In severe preeclampsia, examination of the optic fundi can give an indication of optic vasospasm. Cerebral irritability can be assessed by the degree of hyperreflexia or the presence of clonus (significant if more than three beats).

Fluid balance

The reduced intravascular compartment in preeclampsia, together with poorly controlled fluid balance, can result in circulatory overload, pulmonary oedema, acute respiratory distress syndrome and ultimately death. In severe preeclampsia a central venous pressure (CVP) line may be considered; measurements are taken hourly. If the value is >10 mmHg, then 20 mg furosemide should be considered. Intravenous fluids are administered using infusion pumps; the total recommended fluid intake in severe preeclampsia is 85 mL/h.

Oxytocin should be administered with caution, as it has an antidiuretic effect.

Urinary output should be monitored and urinalysis undertaken every 4 hours to detect the presence of protein, ketones and glucose.

In severe preeclampsia a urinary catheter should be in situ and urine output is measured hourly; a level >30 mL/h reflects adequate renal function.

Plasma volume expansion

Although women with preeclampsia have oedema, they are hypovolaemic. The blood volume of women with preeclampsia is reduced, as shown by a high haemoglobin (Hb) concentration and a high haematocrit level. This results in movement of fluid into the extravascular compartment, causing oedema. The oedema initially occurs in dependent tissues, but as the disease progresses oedema occurs in the liver and brain.

Pain relief

Epidural analgesia may procure the best pain relief, reduce the blood pressure and facilitate rapid caesarean section, should the need arise. It is important to ensure a normal clotting screen and a platelet count >100×10^9/L prior to insertion of the epidural.

Fetal condition

The fetal heart rate should be monitored closely. Deviations from the normal must be reported and acted upon.

Birth plan

When the second stage commences, the obstetrician and paediatrician should be notified. A short second stage may be prescribed, depending on the maternal and fetal conditions. If the maternal or fetal condition shows significant deterioration during the first stage of labour, a caesarean section will be undertaken.

Oxytocin is the preferred agent for the management of the third stage of labour.

Ergometrine and syntometrine will cause peripheral vasoconstriction and increase hypertension; they should therefore not normally be used in the presence of any degree of preeclampsia, unless there is severe haemorrhage.

Postpartum care

The maternal condition should continue to be monitored at least every 4 hours for the next 24 hours or more following childbirth, as there is still a potential danger of the mother developing eclampsia.

Signs of impending eclampsia

- A sharp rise in blood pressure
- Diminished urinary output
- Increase in proteinuria
- Headache, which is usually severe, persistent and frontal in location
- Drowsiness or confusion
- Visual disturbances, such as blurring of vision or flashing lights
- Epigastric pain
- Nausea and vomiting

The aim of care at this time is to prevent death of the mother and fetus by controlling hypertension, inhibiting convulsions and preventing coma.

Further reading

Action on pre-eclampsia (APEC), 2004. PRECOG: The preeclampsia community guideline. http://action-on-pre-eclampsia.org.uk/wp-content/uploads/2012/07/PRECOG-Community-Guideline.pdf.

Continued

Further reading—cont'd

Action on pre-eclampsia, 2004.[a] e-learning package for midwives.
   http://action-on-pre-eclampsia.org.uk/professional-area/
   midwives-e-learning-presentation/.
National Institute for Health and Care Excellence, 2010, updated 2011.
   Hypertension in pregnancy: diagnosis and management. Clinical
   guideline 107. https://www.nice.org.uk/guidance/cg107.
Payne, J., 2016. Pre-eclampsia and eclampsia. Professional reference.
   http://patient.info/doctor/pre-eclampsia-and-eclampsia.

[a]This e-learning resource is currently being updated and a new version is expected shortly.

Prematurity/preterm birth

Prematurity is defined as birth occurring before the end of the 37th gestational week, regardless of birth weight. Most preterm babies are appropriately grown; some are small for gestational age (SGA), while a small number are large for gestational age (LGA), mostly where the mother has diabetes.

Causes of preterm labour

Spontaneous causes

- Forty percent unknown
- Multiple gestation
- Hyperpyrexia as a result of viral or bacterial infection
- Premature rupture of the membranes caused by maternal infection
- Maternal short stature
- Maternal age and parity
- Poor obstetric history; history of preterm labour
- Cervical incompetence
- Poor social circumstances

Elective causes

- Pregnancy-induced hypertension, preeclampsia, chronic hypertension
- Maternal disease: renal, cardiac
- Placenta praevia, abruptio placenta
- Rhesus incompatibility
- Congenital abnormality
- Intrauterine growth restriction

Appearance of the preterm baby

+ Posture appears flattened with hips abducted, knees and ankles flexed
+ Babies are generally hypotonic with a weak and feeble cry
+ Head is in proportion to the body
+ The skull bones are soft with large fontanelles and wide sutures
+ Chest is small and narrow and appears underdeveloped due to minimal lung expansion during fetal life
+ Abdomen is prominent because the liver and spleen are large and abdominal muscle tone is poor
+ Umbilicus appears low in the abdomen because linear growth is cephalocaudal (more apparent nearer to the head than the feet)
+ Subcutaneous fat is laid down from 28 weeks' gestation; therefore, its presence and abundance will affect the redness and transparency of the skin
+ Vernix caseosa is abundant in the last trimester and tends to accumulate at sites of dense lanugo growth, i.e., face, ears, shoulders, sacral region
+ Ear pinna is flat with little curve, the eyes bulge, the orbital ridges are prominent
+ Nipple areola is poorly developed and barely visible
+ Cord is white, fleshy and glistening
+ Plantar creases are absent before 36 weeks
+ In girls, the labia majora fail to cover the labia minora; in boys, the testes descend into the scrotal sac in about the 37th gestational week

Management at birth

+ Current cot availability in the neonatal intensive care unit (NICU), transitional care unit (as applicable) and postnatal ward should be known.
+ The ambient temperature of the birthing room should ideally be between 23°C and 25°C.
+ The neonatal resuscitaire should be checked and ready for use.
+ A second person skilled in resuscitation skills should be present.
+ On cutting the cord, leave an extra length, in case access to the umbilical vessels is necessary later.
+ The Apgar score is traditionally scored at 1 and 5 minutes.
+ Labelling of the preterm/low birth weight (LBW) baby is particularly important because separation of mother and baby could happen at any time if the baby's condition becomes unstable.
+ A detailed but expedient examination of the baby should be carried out.
+ Once it is established that the baby is healthy, the midwife may attempt to normalize care by emphasizing to the parents the importance of

preventing cold stress and promoting skin-to-skin contact for a period of up to 50 minutes.

+ Ensure that the baby is thoroughly dried before skin-to-skin contact is attempted.
+ The baby's body temperature should be maintained between 36.5°C and 37.3°C.

Thermoregulation

Thermoregulation is the balance between heat production and heat loss. The prevention of cold stress, which may lead to hypothermia (body temperature <36°C), is critical. Newborn babies are unable to shiver, move very much or ask for an extra blanket, and therefore rely upon physical adaptations that generate heat by raising their basal metabolic rate and utilizing brown fat deposits. As body temperature falls, tissue oxygen consumption rises as the baby attempts to raise its metabolic rate by burning glucose to generate energy and heat. Care measures should aim to provide an environment that supports thermoneutrality.

+ All preterm babies are prone to heat loss because their ability to produce heat is compromised by their immaturity, so factors like their large surface area to weight ratio, their varying amounts of subcutaneous fat and their ability to mobilize brown fat stores will be affected by their gestational age.
+ During cooling, the immature heat-regulating centres in the hypothalamus and medulla oblongata fail, to different degrees, to recognize and marshal adequately coordinated homeostatic controls.
+ Preterm babies are often unable to increase their oxygen consumption effectively through normal respiratory function, and their calorific intake is often inadequate to meet increasing metabolic requirements.
+ Their open resting postures increase their surface area and insensible water losses.
+ Babies under 2.0 kg may need incubator care when the baby is not in skin-to-skin contact with either parent. The warm conditions in an incubator can be achieved either by heating the air to 30–32°C (air mode) or by servo-controlling the baby's body temperature at a desired set point (36°C). In servo mode, a thermocouple is taped to the upper abdomen and the incubator heater maintains the skin at that site to a preset constant. Babies are clothed with bedding, in a room temperature of 26°C.
+ Most preterm babies between 2.0 and 2.5 kg will be cared for in a cot, in a room temperature of 24°C.

Hypoglycaemia

Low blood glucose concentration is more likely to occur in conditions where babies become cold or where the initiation of early feeding (within the first hour) is delayed.

+ The aim is to maintain the true blood sugar above 2.6 mmol/dL.
+ The preterm baby may be sleepier, and attempts to take the first feed may reflect gestational age.
+ Total feed requirements (60 mL/kg on the first day, with 30 mL/kg increments per day thereafter) may not be taken directly from the breast and supplementary feeds can be given by cup.

Both preterm and SGA babies benefit from human milk because it contains long-chain polyunsaturated omega 3 fatty acids, which are thought to be essential for the myelination of neural membranes and retinal development. Preterm breast milk has:

+ a higher concentration of lipids, protein, sodium, calcium and immunoglobulins
+ low osmolarity
+ lipases and enzymes that improve digestion and absorption

The baby is normally able to coordinate breathing with sucking and swallowing reflexes between 32 and 36 weeks. Preterm babies are limited in their ability to suck by their weak musculature and flexor control, which is important for firm lip and jaw closure. Before 32 weeks, most healthy preterm babies will need to be tube-fed on a regular basis, usually on a 3-hourly regime with breast milk or formula milk.

The care environment

The ideal environment should provide a cycle of day and night, regular nourishment, rest, stimulation and loving attention. The mother's desire to be involved is seen as an *essential* element in the success of caring for LBW babies on postnatal wards.

Handling and touch

Kangaroo care (KC) is used to promote closeness between a baby and mother and involves placing the nappy-clad baby upright between the maternal breasts for skin-to-skin contact, for varying periods of time that suit the mother (can also be carried out by fathers).

Noise and light hazards

+ Noise should be kept to a minimum
+ In dimmed lighting conditions, preterm babies are more able to improve their quality of sleep and alert status

- Reduced light levels at night will help to promote the development of circadian rhythms and diurnal cycles
- Screens to shield adjacent babies from phototherapy lights are essential

Sleeping position

Preterm babies have reduced muscle power and bulk, with flaccid muscle tone; therefore, their movements are erratic, weak or flailing. Without support they may, to differing degrees, develop head, shoulder and hip flattening, which in turn can lead to poor mobility. Nesting the more immature preterm babies into soft bedding, in addition to the use of close flexible boundaries, helps to keep their limbs in midline flexion. However, it is vital that they are nursed in a supine position to prevent asphyxia.

Sudden infant death syndrome (SIDS)

There is a need to remind parents constantly of the risk factors and safety procedures (feet-to-foot sleeping position, smoke-free room) associated with SIDS, alongside teaching them to keep their babies warm while ensuring that they do not overheat them. The midwife needs to explain that families should take into consideration time of year, gestational age and postnatal age. Parental training on 'what to do if my baby stops breathing' should be offered to parents but the decision to receive training should be their choice.

The prevention of infection

LBW babies, particularly preterm ones, are especially vulnerable to infections caused by immaturity of their host defence systems.

Further reading

NHS Choices, 2015. Pregnancy and baby: premature labour and birth. http://www.nhs.uk/conditions/pregnancy-and-baby/pages/premature-early-labour.aspx.

Institute of Medicine (US), 2007. Preterm birth: causes, consequences, and prevention. http://www.ncbi.nlm.nih.gov/pubmed/20669423.

World Health Organization, 2015. Preterm birth. http://www.who.int/mediacentre/factsheets/fs363/en/.

Prostaglandins

A group of compounds with hormone-like effects, notably the production of uterine contractions. A low-dose prostaglandin can be used to bring about effacement and dilation of the cervix without stimulating contractions, and also in the induction of labour in postterm pregnancy. They are used in termination of pregnancy in the second trimester, accompanied by large doses of oxytocin.

Puerperal psychosis

Puerperal psychosis is a serious psychiatric disorder that develops during the perinatal period. It is the most severe form of postpartum affective disorder. The onset is very sudden, the majority presenting in the first 14 days postpartum, most commonly between day 3 and day 7.

Features may include:

+ restlessness and agitation
+ confusion and perplexity
+ suspicion and fear, even terror
+ insomnia
+ episodes of mania making the woman hyperactive (e.g., talking rapidly and incessantly, and being very overactive and elated)
+ neglect of basic needs (e.g., nutrition and hydration)
+ hallucinations and morbid delusional thoughts involving self and baby
+ major behavioural disturbance
+ profound depressive mood

Care and management should be based on:

+ preventive measures preconception/antenatally
+ interprofessional collaboration
+ care in a specialist mother and baby unit

Further reading

National Institute of Health and Care Excellence, 2014, updated 2015. Antenatal and postnatal mental health: clinical management and service guidance. Clinical guideline 192. https://www.nice.org.uk/guidance/cg192.

Royal College of Psychiatrists, 2014. Postpartum psychosis: severe mental illness after childbirth. http://www.rcpsych.ac.uk/healthadvice/problemsdisorders/postpartumpsychosis.aspx.

Pyrexia

Pyrexia is defined as a body temperature above the normal range (34.6–37.6°C). It is a common sign of bacterial or viral infection, and can be an important early indication of serious infection, including puerperal sepsis, chorioamnionitis, wound infection, breast infection, pyelonephritis, pneumonia or subacute bacterial endocarditis, which may lead to systemic sepsis causing significant maternal morbidity and maternal and fetal mortality.

In labour, the most common causes of pyrexia are maternal dehydration, chorioamnionitis and effects of epidural anaesthesia. The Modified Early Obstetric Warning Scoring (MEOWS) system charts should be used to ensure timely recognition, treatment and referral of the woman who may have, or be developing, a critical illness.

Temperature control

+ Paracetamol 1g given orally or intravenously may be used to reduce pyrexia, although the possibility of masking underlying sepsis should not be overlooked
+ Intravenous rehydration may be required if the woman shows signs of dehydration
+ If temperature remains at ≥38.0°C for 30 minutes, antibiotics should be initiated and blood cultures should be taken to investigate potential infection

Pyrexia in neonates

Early-onset neonatal bacterial infection (infection with onset within 72 hours of birth) is a significant cause of mortality and morbidity in newborn babies. Parent organizations and the scientific literature report that there can be unnecessary delays in recognizing and treating sick babies. In addition, concern about the possibility of early-onset neonatal infection is common. This concern is an important influence on the care given to pregnant women and newborn babies. There is wide variation in how the risk of early-onset neonatal infection is managed in healthy babies. The approach taken needs to

+ prioritize the treatment of sick babies
+ minimize the impact of management pathways on healthy women and babies
+ use antibiotics wisely to avoid the development of resistance to antibiotics.

Parents and carers whose babies are at risk of or have an early-onset neonatal infection should have the opportunity to make informed decisions about their baby's, and their own, care and treatment, in partnership with their healthcare professionals.

Sometimes if a baby appears to have a serious illness that could indicate the need for urgent treatment the medical staff may not have time to fully discuss what is involved in that treatment beforehand. In an emergency, if the person with parental responsibility cannot be contacted, healthcare professionals may give treatment immediately if it is in the baby's best interests.

Further reading

Chen, K.T., 2016. Intrapartum fever. http://www.uptodate.com/contents/intrapartum-fever.

National Institute for Health and Care Excellence, 2012. Neonatal infection: antibiotics for prevention and treatment. Clinical guideline CG149. https://www.nice.org.uk/guidance/cg149.

Polin, R.A., 2012. Management of neonates with suspected or proven early-onset bacterial sepsis. Committee on Fetus and Newborn (American Academy of Pediatrics). Pediatrics 129, 5. http://pediatrics.aappublications.org/content/129/5/1006.

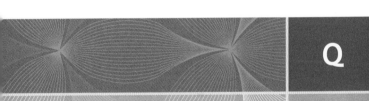

Q

Quadruplets

A quadruple pregnancy is a multiple pregnancy in which four fetuses develop in the uterus at the same time. Quadruplets are extremely rare in the UK, at around 1 in 700,000 pregnancies, although the incidence is higher in other parts of the world, e.g., West Africa. When in vitro fertilization (IVF) treatments were first introduced, with no limit to the number of embryos that could be implanted, the incidence of multiple pregnancies—quadruplets, quintuplets, sextuplets and septuplets—increased, but survival rates in these pregnancies were low.

See also Multiple pregnancies.

Quickening

Recognition of fetal movements by the woman in early pregnancy. The first movements of the fetus are felt at around 20 weeks' gestation in a first pregnancy and at around 18 weeks in subsequent pregnancies, although some women experience fetal movements earlier in their pregnancy.

Resuscitation of the newborn

The aims of resuscitation are to:

+ establish and maintain a clear airway, by ventilation and oxygenation
+ ensure effective circulation
+ correct acidosis
+ prevent hypothermia, hypoglycaemia and haemorrhage

As soon as the baby is born, the clock timer should be started. The Apgar score is assessed in the normal manner at 1 minute. In the absence of any respiratory effort, resuscitation measures are commenced (Table 6). The baby's upper airways may be cleared by gentle suction of the oropharynx and nasopharynx and the presence of a heartbeat verified. The baby is dried quickly, transferred to a well-lit resuscitaire and placed on a flat, firm surface at a comfortable working height and under a radiant heat source to prevent hypothermia. The baby's shoulders may be elevated on a small towel, which causes slight extension of the head and straightens the trachea. Hyperextension may cause airway obstruction owing to the short neck of the neonate and large, ill-supported tongue.

Stimulation

Rough handling of the baby merely serves to increase shock and is unnecessary. Gentle stimulation by drying the baby may initiate breathing.

Warmth

Hypothermia exacerbates hypoxia, as essential oxygen and glucose are diverted from the vital centres in order to create heat for survival. Wet towels are removed and the baby's body and head should be covered with a

Table 6 Resuscitation action plan

A	Anticipation	Assessment (Apgar)	Airway—clear debris
B	Breathing	Bag + mask	
C	Circulation	Cardiac massage	Caring—warmth, comfort
D	Doctor	Drugs	Documentation
E	Explanation	Environment	Endotracheal tube
F	Follow-up care	Family	

prewarmed blanket, leaving only the chest exposed. *Note that it is hazardous to use a silver swaddler under a radiant heater because it could cause burning.*

Clearing the airway

Most babies require no airway clearance at birth; however, if there is obvious respiratory difficulty a suction catheter may be used (size 10 FG, or 8 FG in preterm). The catheter tip should not be inserted further than 5 cm and each suction attempt should not last longer than 5 seconds. Even with a soft catheter, it is still possible to traumatize the delicate mucosa, especially in the preterm baby.

If meconium is present in the airway, suction under direct vision should be performed by the passage of a laryngoscope blade and visualizing the larynx. Care should be taken to avoid touching the vocal cords, as this may induce laryngospasm, apnoea and bradycardia. Thick meconium may need to be aspirated out of the trachea through an endotracheal tube.

Ventilation and oxygenation

If the baby fails to respond to these simple measures, assisted ventilation is necessary.

Facemask ventilation

+ An appropriately sized mask (usually 00 or 0/1) is positioned on the face so that it covers the nose and mouth and ensures a good seal.
+ A 500-mL bag is used, as a smaller 250-mL bag does not permit sustained inflation.
+ Care should be taken not to apply pressure on the soft tissue under the jaw, as this may obstruct the airway.
+ To aerate the lungs five sustained inflations are delivered, using oxygen or air or a combination of both, with a pressure of 30 cmH$_2$O (water pressure) applied for 2–3 seconds and repeated five times; then continue to ventilate at a rate of 40 respirations per minute. Only continue on to ventilation respirations if chest movement is achieved. If chest movement is not achieved reposition and repeat the five inflation breaths.
+ Insertion of a neonatal airway helps to prevent obstruction by the baby's tongue.
+ Note that overextension of the baby's head causes airway obstruction. A longer inspiration phase improves oxygenation. Higher inflation pressures may be required to produce chest movement.

Endotracheal intubation

If the baby fails to respond to intermittent positive pressure ventilation (IPPV) by bag and mask, or if bradycardia is present, an endotracheal tube should be passed without delay. Intubating a baby requires special skill that, once acquired, must be practised if it is to be retained.

Technique for intubation

+ Position the baby on a flat surface, preferably a resuscitaire, and extend the neck into the 'neutral position'. A rolled-up towel placed under the shoulders will help maintain proper alignment.
+ The blade of the laryngoscope is introduced over the baby's tongue into the pharynx until the epiglottis is seen.
+ Elevation of the epiglottis with the tip of the laryngoscope reveals the vocal cords.
+ Any mucus, blood or meconium which is obstructing the trachea should be cleared by careful suction prior to passing the endotracheal tube a distance of 1.5–2 cm into the trachea. (Pressure on the cricoid cartilage may facilitate visualization of the larynx.)
+ Intubation may be easier if a tracheal introducer made of plastic-covered soft metal wire is used. This will increase the stiffness and curvature of the tube.
+ After the laryngoscope is removed, oxygen is administered by IPPV to the endotracheal tube via the Ambu bag. A maximum of 30 cmH$_2$O should be applied, as there is risk of rupture of alveoli or tension pneumothorax with higher pressures.

The rise and fall of the chest wall should indicate whether the tube is in the trachea. This can be confirmed by auscultation of the chest. Distension of the stomach indicates oesophageal intubation, necessitating re-siting of the tube.

Mouth-to-face/nose resuscitation

In the absence of specialized equipment, assisted ventilation can be achieved by mouth-to-face resuscitation.

+ With the baby's head in the 'sniffing' position, the operator places his/her mouth over the baby's mouth and nose.
+ Using only the air in her buccal cavity, he/she breathes gently into the baby's airway at a rate of 20–30 breaths per minute, allowing the infant to exhale between breaths.

It may be easier with larger babies to use mouth-to-face resuscitation.

External cardiac massage

Chest compressions should be performed if the heart rate is less than 60 beats/min, or between 60 and 100 beats/min and falling despite adequate ventilation. The most effective way of performing chest compressions is to:

- encircle the baby's chest with your fingers on the baby's spine and your thumbs on the lower mid-sternum;
- depress the chest at a rate of 100–120 times per minute, at a ratio of three compressions to one ventilation, and at a depth of one-third (2–3 cm) of the baby's chest.

(Excessive pressure over the lower end of the sternum may cause rib, lung or liver damage.)

Use of drugs

If the baby's response is slow or he/she remains hypotonic after ventilation is achieved, consideration will be given to the use of drugs. In specialist obstetric units, pulse oximetry may be employed to monitor hypoxia and can be blood obtained through the umbilical artery or vein to ascertain biochemical status. Results will enable appropriate administration of resuscitation drugs:

Naloxone hydrochloride

Naloxone is a powerful antiopioid drug for the reversal of the effects of maternal narcotic drugs given in the preceding 3 hours. It should be used with caution and only in specific circumstances.

- Ventilation should be established prior to its use.
- It must *not* be given to apnoeic babies.
- A dose of up to 100 µg/kg body weight may be administered intramuscularly for prolonged action.
- As opioid action may persist for some hours, the midwife must be alert for signs of relapse when a repeat dose may be required.
- It should *not* be administered to babies of narcotic-addicted mothers, as this may precipitate acute withdrawal.

Sodium bicarbonate

This is not recommended for brief periods of cardiopulmonary resuscitation.

- Once tissues are oxygenated by lung inflation with 100% oxygen and cardiac compression, the acidosis will self-correct unless asphyxia is very severe.
- If the heart rate is less than 60 beats/min despite effective ventilation, chest compression and two intravenous doses of adrenaline (epinephrine) then sodium bicarbonate 4.2% solution (0.5 mmol/mL) can be administered using 2–4 mL/kg (1–2 mmol/kg) by slow intravenous injection.

* It should be given at a rate of 1 mL/minute in order to avoid rapid elevation of serum osmolality with the attendant risk of intracranial haemorrhage.
* It should *not* be given prior to ventilation being established.
* THAM 7% (*tris*-hydroxymethyl-amino-methane) 0.5 mmol/kg may be used in preference to sodium bicarbonate.

Adrenaline (epinephrine)

This is indicated if the heart rate is less than 60 beats/min despite 1 minute of effective ventilation and chest compression.

* An initial dose of 0.1–0.3 mL/kg of 1:10,000 solution (10–30 μg/kg) can be given intravenously; this may be repeated after 3 minutes for a further two doses.
* The Royal College of Paediatrics and Child Health (1997) recommends a higher dose of 100 μg/kg intravenously, if there is no response to the boluses. It is reasonable to try giving one dose of adrenaline (epinephrine) 0.1 mL/kg of 1:1000 via the endotracheal tube, as this sometimes has an immediate effect.

Hypoglycaemia is not usually a problem unless resuscitation has been prolonged. A solution of dextrose 10% 3 mL/kg may be given intravenously to correct a blood sugar of less than 2.5 mmol/L.

Observations and aftercare

Throughout the resuscitation procedure the baby's response is monitored and recorded. An accurate written record detailing the resuscitation events is essential. The endotracheal tube may be left in place for a few minutes after the baby starts to breathe spontaneously. Suction may be applied through the endotracheal tube as it is removed.

Explanation must be given to the parents about the resuscitation and the need for transfer to hospital (if the baby was born at home) or to the neonatal unit. The principles of resuscitation of the newborn are applicable wherever and whenever apnoea occurs. The midwife must be able to implement emergency care while awaiting medical assistance:

Key points for practice

* Anticipation of problems
* Checking of resuscitation equipment
* Starting clock
* Suctioning
* Keeping baby warm
* Apgar score
* Bag and mask ventilation

- Endotracheal ventilation
- Cardiac massage
- Drugs
- Other problems

Further reading

Wylie, J., Ainsworth, S., Tinnion, R., 2015. Resuscitation Council UK Resuscitation and support of transition of babies at birth. https://www.resus.org.uk/resuscitation-guidelines/ resuscitation-and-support-of-transition-of-babies-at-birth/.

Rhesus D incompatibility

Rhesus D (RhD) isoimmunization causes haemolytic disease of the newborn (HDN). Few antibodies to blood group antigens other than those in the Rh system cause severe HDN; fetal transfusion is unusual for multiple maternal antibody isoimmunization without anti-D. ABO incompatibility (see ABO incompatibility) is possibly the most frequent cause of mild to moderate haemolysis in neonates.

RhD incompatibility can occur when a woman with Rh-negative blood type is pregnant with a fetus with Rh-positive blood type.

- The placenta normally prevents fetal blood entering the maternal circulation. However, during pregnancy or birth, small amounts of fetal Rh-positive blood cross the placenta and enter the circulation of the mother, who has Rh-negative blood.
- The woman's immune system reacts by producing anti-D antibodies that cause sensitization.
- In subsequent pregnancies these maternal antibodies can cross the placenta and destroy fetal erythrocytes.
- Usually, sensitization occurs during the first pregnancy or birth, leading to extensive destruction of fetal red blood cells during subsequent pregnancies.

Rh isoimmunization can result from any procedure or incident where maternal blood leaks across the placenta or from the inadvertent transfusion of Rh-positive blood to the woman.

Prevention of RhD isoimmunization

This is by routine antenatal anti-D immunoglobulin (Ig) prophylaxis, within 72 hours of birth or after any other sensitizing event. Anti-D Ig is a human plasma-based product that prevents the production of anti-D antibodies by the mother.

Administration of anti-D Ig

Anti-D Ig is administered to Rh-negative women who are pregnant with, or have given birth to, a Rh-positive baby. It destroys any fetal cells in the mother's blood before her immune system produces antibodies. The process for nonsensitized women is:

1. Women who are Rh-negative are screened for Rh antibodies (indirect Coombs test). A negative test shows an *absence* of antibodies or sensitization.

2. Blood is retested at 28 weeks of pregnancy. In countries where antenatal prophylaxis is routine (at 28 and 34 weeks' gestation), the first injection of anti-D Ig is given just after this blood sample is taken.

3. Where a policy of routine antenatal anti-D Ig prophylaxis is *not* in place, blood is retested for antibodies at 34 weeks of pregnancy.

4. When anti-D Ig prophylaxis is given at 28 weeks, blood is not retested, as it is difficult to distinguish passive anti-D Ig from immune anti-D.

5. Following the birth, cord blood is tested for confirmation of Rh type, ABO blood group, haemoglobin (Hb) and serum bilirubin levels and the presence of maternal antibodies on fetal red cells (direct Coombs test). Again, a negative test indicates an absence of antibodies or sensitization. The postnatal dose of anti-D Ig is *still given* if passive anti-D Ig is present.

6. A Kleihauer acid elution test is also carried out on an anticoagulated maternal blood sample immediately after birth to estimate the number of fetal cells in a sample of maternal blood.

7. Anti-D Ig must always be given as soon as possible after, and in any case within 72 hours of, any sensitizing event and the birth. Anti-D Ig is injected into the deltoid muscle, from which absorption is optimal.

Dose of anti-D Ig

Research evidence for the optimal dose is still limited but the doses listed below are recommended:

+ 500 IU anti-D Ig at 28 and 34 weeks' gestation for women in their first pregnancy.

+ At least 500 IU for all nonsensitized Rh-negative woman following the birth of a Rh-positive infant.

+ 250 IU following sensitizing events *up to* 20 weeks' gestation.

+ At least 500 IU following sensitizing events *after* 20 weeks' gestation.

+ Larger doses for traumatic events and procedures such as caesarean birth, stillbirths and intrauterine deaths, abdominal trauma during the third trimester, or manual removal of the placenta (dose calculated on 500 IU of anti-D Ig suppressing immunization from 4 mL of RhD-positive red blood cells [RBCs]).

‣ Larger doses for any other instance of inadvertent transfusion of Rh-positive RBCs, e.g., from an incorrect blood transfusion of Rh-positive blood platelets.

Ethical and legal issues

Anti-D Ig is a human plasma-based product. To give informed consent to its use, women need to know the possible consequences of treatment, as opposed to nontreatment, with anti-D Ig.

Management of RhD isoimmunization

Effects of RhD isoimmunization.

‣ Destruction of fetal RBCs results in anaemia, possibly oedema and congestive cardiac failure.

‣ Fetal bilirubin levels also increase as more red cells are destroyed, with possible neurological damage as bilirubin is deposited in the brain.

‣ Lesser degrees of destruction result in haemolytic anaemia, while extensive haemolysis can cause hydrops fetalis and death in utero.

Antenatal monitoring and treatment of RhD isoimmunization

Depending on the severity of Rh isoimmunization, monitoring and treatment can include the following:

‣ Women who are Rh-negative are screened for Rh antibodies (indirect Coombs test). A positive test indicates the *presence* of antibodies or sensitization.

‣ RBCs obtained by chorionic villus sampling (using an immune rosette technique) can be Rh phenotyped as early as 9–11 weeks' gestation.

‣ Maternal blood is retested frequently to monitor any increase in antibody titres. Sudden and unexpected rises in serum anti-D levels can result in hydrops fetalis.

‣ If antibody titres remain stable, ongoing monitoring is continued.

‣ If antibody titres increase, Doppler ultrasonography of the middle cerebral artery peak systolic velocity is used rather than amniocentesis to detect fetal anaemia.

‣ Changes in fetal serum bilirubin levels are observed.

‣ The fetus is closely monitored by ultrasonography for oedema and hepatosplenomegaly.

‣ Intravenous immunoglobulin (IVIG) has the potential to maintain the fetus until intrauterine fetal transfusion (IUT) can be performed. IVIG works by blocking Fc-mediated antibody transport across the placenta, blocking fetal red cell destruction and reducing maternal antibody levels.

- IUT can be used from about 20 weeks of gestation to reduce the effects of haemolysis until the fetus is capable of survival outside the uterus.
- Early delivery depends on the ongoing severity of the haemolysis and the condition of the fetus.

Postnatal treatment of RhD isoimmunization

- Babies with mild to moderate haemolytic anaemia and hyperbilirubinemia may require careful monitoring but less aggressive management.
- Babies with hydrops fetalis are pale and have oedema and ascites; in some cases, they may be stillborn.
- Management of surviving infants aims to prevent further haemolysis, reduce bilirubin levels, remove maternal Rh antibodies from the baby's circulation and combat anaemia.
- In some cases, phototherapy can be effective but exchange transfusion is often required, and packed cell transfusion may be needed to increase Hb levels.
- Infants are at risk of ongoing haemolytic anaemia.
  See also Antenatal care.

Further reading

Gandhi, A., 2016. Haemolytic disease of the fetus and newborn. Professional reference. https://patient.info/doctor/haemolytic-disease-of-the-fetus-and-newborn.

National Institute for Health and Clinical Excellence, 2008. Routine anti-D prophylaxis for women who are rhesus D negative. Technology appraisal 156. https://www.nice.org.uk/guidance/ta156.

Qyreshi, H., Massey, E., Kirwan, D., et al. for the British Committee for Standards in Haematology (BCSH), 2014. BCSH guideline for the use of anti-D immunoglobulin for the prevention of haemolytic disease of the fetus and newborn. Transfus. Med. doi: 10.1111/tme.12091. http://onlinelibrary.wiley.com/doi/10.1111/tme.12091/abstract.

Rubella

Rubella (German measles) is a mild viral infection that is trivial in children, more severe in adults. One attack confers immunity. Maternal rubella infection in early weeks of pregnancy causes fetal damage (commonly multiple defects) in up to 90% of infants. Congenital rubella syndrome (CRS) is a major cause of developmental abnormalities including blindness and deafness. Generally presents with macular facial rash that spreads to trunk and limbs, fading within 4 days; also cervical lymphadenopathy, fever and myalgia. Spread is by airborne droplets. Vaccine given in childhood as part of the triple MMR (measles, mumps and rubella) vaccine.

Midwives should check the woman's rubella immune status as part of routine antenatal care. This is determined by measuring the rubella antibody titre. Women who are not immune should be advised to avoid contact with anyone with rubella, and may wish to discuss termination of the pregnancy if they have already been exposed. Exposure in the first trimester can result in spontaneous abortion. Infection occurring within 11 days of the last menstrual period is unlikely to result in intrauterine infection, and proven infection occurring later in pregnancy (after 16th week) is less likely to result in severe fetal sequelae.

Babies born with CRS are highly infectious and should be isolated from other infants and pregnant women, but not their own mothers.

Vaccination should be offered during the puerperium and subsequent pregnancy avoided for at least 3 months.

Rubin manoeuvre

A rotational manoeuvre to relieve shoulder dystocia. Pressure is exerted over the fetal back to adduct and rotate the shoulders.

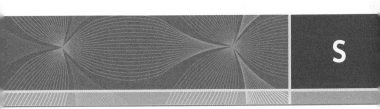

S

Sepsis

Sepsis is a potentially life-threatening condition and a medical emergency. Sepsis may not be obvious and a high index of suspicion is often required to make the diagnosis. Early aggressive treatment increases the chances of survival and every hour that treatment is delayed increases mortality.

See also Shock.

> **Further reading**
>
> Royal College of Obstetricians and Gynaecologists, 2012. Bacterial sepsis in pregnancy. Green-top guideline no 64a. https://www.rcog.org.uk/globalassets/documents/guidelines/gtg_64a.pdf.
>
> Royal College of Obstetricians and Gynaecologists, 2012. Bacterial sepsis following pregnancy. Green-top guideline no. 64b. https://www.rcog.org.uk/globalassets/documents/guidelines/gtg_64b.pdf.
>
> Tidy, C., 2016. Sepsis. Professional reference. http://patient.info/doctor/sepsis-septicaemia-pro.

Sexually transmitted infections

The high rates of, and increase in, sexually transmitted infection (STI) diagnoses, particularly in women aged 16–24, is of concern. Most at risk are those who have high numbers of sexual partners, partner change and unprotected sexual intercourse.

Joint management between an obstetrician and a genitourinary medicine (GUM) physician during pregnancy is essential for women with infections that are serious, life-threatening or both, such as human immunodeficiency virus (HIV); in addition, a paediatrician is required in the care and management of the neonate infected through vertical transmission. The midwife plays a vital role in the provision of individualized care throughout pregnancy, labour and the puerperium.

STIs include:

Trichomoniasis

Caused by infection with the parasite *Trichomonas vaginalis*, a round or oval flagellated protozoan, trichomoniasis can cause vulval pruritus and inflammation. However, 10%–50% of women are asymptomatic.

Trichomoniasis has been linked with a small risk of preterm birth and low birth weight, and an increase in the risk of HIV via sexual intercourse. Trichomoniasis may be acquired perinatally. Diagnosis is usually by cultures. The recommended treatment is metronidazole daily for 5–7 days or as a single dose. It is usual to treat partner(s) and advise against intercourse until treatment is completed.

Bacterial vaginosis

Bacterial vaginosis (BV) is the most common cause of vaginal discharge in women of childbearing age. It can arise and remit spontaneously in sexually active and non-sexually active women. It often coexists with other STIs. BV is present in up to 20% of women during pregnancy, although the majority are asymptomatic. BV during pregnancy is associated with preterm birth, low birth weight, preterm premature rupture of membranes, intraamniotic infection and postpartum endometritis.

Antibiotic therapy is highly effective at eradicating infection and improving the outcome of pregnancy for women with a past history of preterm birth.

Candidiasis

Vaginal candidiasis is found 2–10 times more frequently in pregnant than in non-pregnant women and it is more difficult to eradicate. Treatment is primarily with antifungal pessaries or cream (e.g., clotrimazole). Diflucan is available from pharmacies without a prescription but has not been evaluated in pregnancy and cannot be assumed to be safe. It should also be used with caution whilst breastfeeding owing to toxic effects in high doses.

Bacterial infections
Chlamydia

Chlamydia trachomatis is an intracellular bacterium. It is the most common cause of sexually transmitted bacterial infection and a leading cause of pelvic inflammatory disease (PID).

Chlamydial infection is asymptomatic in approximately 80% of cases. Some women may have a purulent vaginal discharge, postcoital or intermenstrual bleeding, lower abdominal pain, mucopurulent cervicitis and/or contact bleeding. Chlamydial infection of the cervix is found in 15%–30% of women attending GUM clinics. It is found concurrently in 35%–40% of women with gonorrhoea.

Chlamydia in pregnancy
Chlamydia in pregnancy can cause amnionitis and postpartum endometritis.

Fetal and neonatal infections
The major risk to the infant is from passing through an infected cervix during birth. Up to 70% of babies born to mothers with chlamydial infection will become infected, with 30%–40% developing conjunctivitis and 10%–20% a characteristic pneumonia. The incubation period of chlamydial ophthalmia is 6–21 days. Chlamydial pneumonia usually occurs between the 4th and 11th weeks of life. It affects about half of the babies who develop conjunctivitis but is not always preceded by it. The pharynx, middle

ear, rectum and vagina are also targets for infection, with a delay of up to 7 months before cultures become positive.

Genital chlamydial infections are sensitive to three classes of antibiotic—tetracyclines, macrolides (e.g., erythromycin) and the fluorinated quinolones, especially ofloxacin.

The tetracyclines and the fluoroquinolones are currently contraindicated in pregnancy. Erythromycin is the preferred treatment for cervical chlamydial infection despite its gastrointestinal effects. Erythromycin is also used for chlamydial infections in infants, young children and pregnant and lactating women. Single-dose azithromycin is expensive but gaining favour because of its effectiveness, low incidence of adverse gastrointestinal effects and enhanced compliance.

Gonorrhoea

Gonorrhoea is caused by *Neisseria gonorrhoeae*, a gram-negative diplococcus. Transmission is by sexual contact. This organism adheres to mucous membranes. The primary sites of infection are therefore the mucous membranes of the urethra, endocervix, rectum, pharynx and conjunctiva. Gonorrhoea may coexist with other genital mucosal pathogens, notably *Trichomonas vaginalis*, *Candida albicans* and *Candida trachomatis*. Gonorrhoea is a major cause of PID. The sequelae of PID include:

+ infertility
+ ectopic pregnancy
+ chronic pelvic pain

Although uncommon, gonorrhoea may also cause disseminated systemic disease and arthritis. The most common symptom is an increased or altered vaginal discharge, although up to 50% of women are asymptomatic. Lower abdominal pain, dysuria, intermenstrual uterine bleeding and menorrhagia may also be experienced, ranging in intensity from minimal to severe.

Gonorrhoea in pregnancy

The incidence of gonorrhoea in pregnancy is low but its presence has been associated with:

+ spontaneous abortion
+ very low birth weight
+ prelabour rupture of the membranes
+ chorioamnionitis
+ preterm birth
+ postpartum endometritis
+ pelvic sepsis

Fetal and neonatal infections

N. gonorrhoeae can be transmitted during birth, or occasionally *in utero* when there is prolonged rupture of the membranes. The risk of transmission is between 30% and 47%. Infection usually manifests as gonococcal ophthalmia neonatorum, a notifiable condition. A profuse, purulent discharge is usually evident within a few days of birth. It can be diagnosed by microscopy and culture of an eye swab. The eyes may be cleaned with saline but systemic antibiotics are required. If left untreated, the condition will eventually lead to blindness, and occasionally the neonate may develop further infection such as gonococcal arthritis.

Treatment with the antibiotic regimen of penicillin and probenicid remains effective. Oral, single-dose preparations are now most commonly given. In the case of penicillin allergy or penicillin-resistant organisms, spectinomycin or ceftriaxone are also effective.

Syphilis

Syphilis is caused by the bacterium *Treponema pallidum*, a spiral organism (spirochaete), and is usually acquired by sexual contact. It can also be congenitally transmitted. It is a complex systemic disease that can involve virtually any organ in the body.

Syphilis in pregnancy

Although sequelae are dependent on the stage of infection in the mother, untreated syphilis in pregnancy may result in:

+ spontaneous abortion
+ preterm birth
+ stillbirth
+ neonatal death
+ significant infant or later morbidity

Vertical transmission may occur at any time during pregnancy, but is more likely if the mother has primary, secondary or early latent syphilis. The infection does not usually occur before the 4th month of pregnancy because treponemes from the maternal circulation are unable to pass through the Langhans cell layer of the early placenta.

Congenital syphilis

Approximately two-thirds of live-born infected infants do not have any signs or symptoms at birth, but they present over the following weeks, months or years. Lesions develop only after the 4th month when immunological competence becomes established. Serology at birth is unreliable owing to passive transfer from the mother and the treponemal-specific immunoglobulin M (IgM) test is prone to false positive and negative results.

Diagnosis

Women in the UK are screened for syphilis at antenatal booking and treated if need be. However, this does not detect women who acquire the infection during pregnancy, or women who are incubating syphilis at the time of serological testing. A range of serological tests is used for screening.

Treatment

The preferred treatment is intramuscular penicillin. In the case of penicillin allergy, the alternative is erythromycin, as tetracycline is contraindicated in pregnancy. The poor placental transfer of erythromycin does not reliably cure the fetus and as a precaution the baby may be given a course of penicillin at birth.

Viral infections

Genital warts

Genital warts are caused by human papillomavirus (HPV) types 6 and 11. Transmission is most often by sexual contact, although infants and young children may develop laryngeal papillomas after being infected from maternal genital warts at birth.

In pregnancy, genital warts may dramatically increase in size and appear as cauliflower-like masses, although they usually diminish in size following the birth. Occasionally they can obstruct a vaginal birth; therefore a caesarean section would be indicated.

- Genital warts are difficult and time-consuming to treat.
- They are usually treated initially with locally applied caustic agents such as podophyllum. However, this is contraindicated in pregnancy because of possible teratogenic effects.
- It is recommended that no treatment be offered during pregnancy, although there are alternatives such as trichloroacetic acid, cryotherapy or electrocautery.

Women presenting with genital warts should be fully investigated to exclude other STIs. In addition, colposcopy should be performed to exclude flat warts on the cervix. Most genital warts are benign, but cervical intraepithelial neoplasia is strongly associated with HPV types 16, 18, 31, 33 and 35; therefore an annual cervical smear is recommended.

Hepatitis

See Hepatitis.

Shock

Shock can be classified as follows:

* *hypovolaemic*—the result of a reduction in intravascular volume
* *cardiogenic*—impaired ability of the heart to pump blood
* *distributive*—an abnormality in the vascular system that produces a maldistribution of the circulatory system; this includes septic shock and anaphylactic shock

Hypovolaemic shock

This is caused by any loss of circulating fluid volume that is not compensated for, as in haemorrhage, but may also occur when there is severe vomiting. The body reacts to the loss of circulating fluid in stages.

Initial stage

The reduction in fluid or blood decreases the venous return to the heart. The ventricles of the heart are inadequately filled, causing a reduction in stroke volume and cardiac output. As cardiac output and venous return fall, the blood pressure is reduced. The drop in blood pressure decreases the supply of oxygen to the tissues and cell function is affected.

Compensatory stage

The drop in cardiac output produces a response from the sympathetic nervous system through the activation of receptors in the aorta and carotid arteries. Blood is redistributed to the vital organs. Vessels in the gastrointestinal tract, kidneys, skin and lungs constrict. This response is seen as the skin becomes pale and cool. Peristalsis slows, urinary output is reduced and exchange of gas in the lungs is impaired as blood flow diminishes. The heart rate increases in an attempt to improve cardiac output and blood pressure. The pupils of the eyes dilate. The sweat glands are stimulated and the skin becomes moist and clammy. Adrenaline (epinephrine) is released from the adrenal medulla and aldosterone from the adrenal cortex. Antidiuretic hormone is secreted from the posterior lobe of the pituitary. Their combined effect is to cause vasoconstriction, an increased cardiac output and a decrease in urinary output. Venous return to the heart will increase but, unless the fluid loss is replaced, will not be sustained.

Progressive stage

This stage leads to multisystem failure. Compensatory mechanisms begin to fail, with vital organs lacking adequate perfusion. Volume depletion causes a further fall in blood pressure and cardiac output. The coronary arteries suffer lack of supply. Peripheral circulation is poor, with weak or absent pulses.

Final, irreversible stage of shock

Multisystem failure and cell destruction are irreparable. Death ensues.

Management

Priorities in the management of hypovolaemic shock:

*   Call for help.
    *   Shock is a progressive condition and delay in correcting hypovolaemia can ultimately lead to maternal death.
*   Maintain the airway.
    *   If the mother is severely collapsed, she should be turned on to her side and 40% oxygen administered at a rate of 4–6 L/min.
    *   If she is unconscious, an airway should be inserted.
*   Replace fluids.
    *   Two wide-bore intravenous cannulae should be inserted to enable fluids and drugs to be administered swiftly.
    *   Blood should be taken for cross-matching prior to commencing intravenous fluids.
    *   A crystalloid solution such as Hartmann solution or Ringer lactate is given until the woman's condition has improved.
    *   To maintain intravascular volume, colloids (e.g., Gelofusine, Haemaccel) are recommended.
*   Ensure warmth.
    *   It is important to keep the woman warm, but not overwarmed or warmed too quickly, as this will cause peripheral vasodilatation and result in hypotension.
*   Arrest haemorrhage.
    *   The source of the bleeding needs to be identified and stopped.
*   Monitor vital signs.

Septic shock

The most common form of sepsis in childbearing in the UK is reported to be that caused by beta-haemolytic *Streptococcus pyogenes* (Lancefield group A). This is a gram-positive organism, responding to intravenous antibiotics, specifically those that are penicillin based. In the general population, infections from gram-negative organisms such as *Escherichia coli*, *Proteus* or *Pseudomonas pyocyaneus* are predominant; these are common pathogens in the female genital tract.

The placental site is the main point of entry for an infection associated with pregnancy and childbirth. This may occur following prolonged rupture of fetal membranes, obstetric trauma or septic abortion, or in the presence of retained placental tissue. Endotoxins present in the organisms release components that trigger the body's immune response, culminating in multiple organ failure.

Clinical presentation

The mother may present with a sudden onset of tachycardia, pyrexia, rigors and tachypnoea. She may also exhibit a change in her mental state. Signs of shock, including hypotension, develop as the condition takes hold. Haemorrhage may develop as a result of disseminated intravascular coagulation.

Management

This is based on preventing further deterioration by restoring circulatory volume and eradication of the infection.

+ Replacement of fluid volume will restore perfusion of the vital organs.
+ Satisfactory oxygenation is also needed.
+ Rigorous treatment with intravenous antibiotics, after blood cultures have been taken, is necessary to halt the illness.
+ Retained products of conception can be detected on ultrasound, and these can then be removed.

Shoulder dystocia

Shoulder dystocia (Fig. 31) is the failure of the shoulders to traverse the pelvis spontaneously after delivery of the head. Incidence is around 0.3% of all deliveries. The anterior shoulder becomes trapped behind or on the symphysis pubis, while the posterior shoulder may be in the hollow of the sacrum or high above the sacral promontory. This is, therefore, a bony dystocia, and traction at this point will further impact the anterior shoulder, impeding attempts at delivery.

Risk factors

These can only give a high index of suspicion:

+ post-term pregnancy
+ high parity
+ maternal obesity (weight over 90 kg)
+ fetal macrosomia (birth weight over 4000 g)
+ maternal diabetes and gestational diabetes
+ prolonged labour (first and second stages)
+ operative delivery

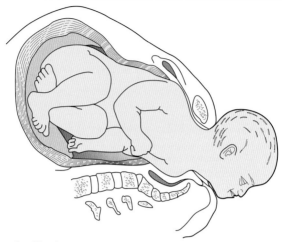

Fig. 31 Shoulder dystocia.

Warning signs and diagnosis

The birth may have been uncomplicated initially, but the head may have advanced slowly and the chin may have had difficulty in sweeping over the perineum. Once the head is born, it may look as if it is trying to return into the vagina.

Shoulder dystocia is diagnosed when manoeuvres normally used by the midwife fail to accomplish birth.

Management

+ Summon help—an obstetrician, an anaesthetist and a person proficient in neonatal resuscitation.
+ Attempt to disimpact the shoulders and accomplish delivery. An accurate and detailed record of the type of manoeuvre(s) used, the time taken, the amount of force used and the outcome of each attempted manoeuvre should be made.
+ Try the procedures for 30–60 seconds; if the baby is not born, move on to the next procedure.

Noninvasive procedures

Change in maternal position

+ McRoberts manoeuvre. Help the woman to lie flat and to bring her knees up to her chest as far as possible to rotate the angle of the symphysis pubis superiorly and use the weight of her legs to create

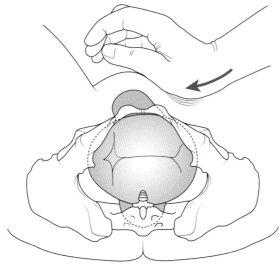

Fig. 32 Suprapubic pressure procedure.

gentle pressure on her abdomen, releasing the impaction of the anterior shoulder

+ Suprapubic pressure. Pressure is exerted on the side of the fetal back and towards the fetal chest to adduct the shoulders and push the anterior shoulder away from the symphysis pubis (Fig. 32). Can be used with the McRoberts manoeuvre.

Manipulative procedures

Where noninvasive procedures have not been successful, direct manipulation of the fetus must now be attempted:

+ *Positioning of the mother.* McRoberts or the all-fours position may be used.
+ *Episiotomy.* May be necessary to gain access to the fetus and reduce maternal trauma.
+ *Rubin manoeuvre.* The posterior shoulder is pushed in the direction of the fetal chest, thus rotating the anterior shoulder away from the symphysis pubis into the oblique diameter.
+ *Wood manoeuvre.* A hand is inserted into the vagina, pressure is exerted on the posterior fetal shoulder, and rotation is achieved.
+ *Reverse Wood manoeuvre.* Fingers on the back of the posterior shoulder apply pressure to rotate in opposite direction.

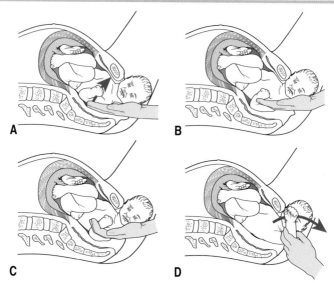

A   **B**

C   **D**

Fig. 33 Delivery of the posterior arm. (A) Location of the posterior arm. (B) Directing the arm into the hollow of the sacrum. (C) Grasping and splinting the wrist and forearm. (D) Sweeping the arm over the chest and delivering the hand.

- *Delivery of the posterior arm.* A hand is inserted into the vagina, and two fingers splint the humerus of the posterior arm, flex the elbow and sweep the forearm over the chest to deliver the hand (Fig. 33). If the rest of the delivery is not then accomplished, the second arm can be delivered following rotation of the shoulder using either Wood or Rubin manoeuvre or by reversing the Løvset manoeuvre. Has a high complication rate.
- *Zavanelli manoeuvre.* If the manoeuvres described above have been unsuccessful, the obstetrician may consider the Zavanelli manoeuvre. Requires the reversal of the mechanisms of delivery so far and success rates vary.

The 'HELPERR' mnemonic is widely used in obstetric drills:
- **H**elp
- **E**pisiotomy need assessed
- **L**egs in McRoberts position
- **P**ressure suprapubically
- **E**nter vagina (internal rotation)
- **R**emove posterior arm
- **R**oll over and try again

Complications associated with shoulder dystocia

+ Postpartum haemorrhage
+ Uterine rupture
+ Neonatal asphyxia
+ Erb palsy
+ Intrauterine death

Further reading

Payne, J., 2016. Dystocia. Professional reference. http://patient.info/doctor/dystocia.

Perinatal Institute. Perinatal review—obstetric emergencies: shoulder dystocia. http://www.perinatal.nhs.uk/reviews/oe/oe_shoulder_dystocia.htm.

Royal College of Obstetricians and Gynaecologists, 2012. Shoulder dystocia. Green-top guideline no. 42. https://www.rcog.org.uk/globalassets/documents/guidelines/gtg_42.pdf.

Smoking in pregnancy

Smoking in pregnancy poses significant health risks to the mother and baby. In addition to all the health risks associated with smoking for the general population, some risks to the mother are specific to pregnancy, including ectopic pregnancy, placenta praevia, and preeclampsia. Pregnant women who smoke are also at increased risk of deep vein thrombosis.

Risks to the fetus are also increased in women who smoke: these include spontaneous abortion, miscarriage, stillbirth, premature birth, low birth weight, intrauterine growth restriction and neonatal death. Babies born to mothers who smoke are also twice as likely to die from sudden unexplained death in infancy. Children of mothers who smoke are more likely to have behavioural problems, learning difficulties, reduced educational performance and are at increased risk of respiratory disease and other upper respiratory tract infections.

Although some women will stop smoking before becoming pregnant or as soon as they know they are pregnant, others will need considerable support to quit. Nicotine in cigarettes is highly addictive and smoking is a chronic relapsing condition.

Midwives have an important role to play in encouraging women to stop smoking in pregnancy (and to quit permanently) and offering very brief advice on smoking has been shown to be effective. The midwife should offer referrals to local Stop Smoking services, and discuss the use of nicotine replacement therapy with women who are having difficulty in quitting. Carbon monoxide screening (to detect smoking) should be carried out routinely on all pregnant women.

Further reading

National Institute for Health and Care Excellence, 2010. Smoking: stopping in pregnancy and after childbirth. Public health guidance 26. https://www.nice.org.uk/guidance/ph26.

NHS Smokefree. Pregnancy and smoking. http://www.nhs.uk/smokefree/why-quit/smoking-in-pregnancy.

Public Health England. National Centre for Smoking Cessation and Training, 2016. Smoking cessation: a briefing for midwifery staff. Third edition. http://www.ncsct.co.uk/usr/pub/Midwifery _briefing_ %20V3.pdf.

Stillbirth

Stillbirth is the term for the death of a baby after 24 weeks of pregnancy but before birth. The legal definition stipulates that the baby should not, 'at any time after being completely expelled from its mother, breathe or show any other sign of life'. A medical practitioner or midwife present at the birth may write and sign a stillbirth certificate. In the UK, registration of the stillbirth must be undertaken before a certificate for burial or cremation can be issued.

See also Intrauterine death.

Symphysiotomy

Symphysiotomy is a surgical procedure to divide the cartilage of the pubic symphysis to widen the pelvis to facilitate delivery of the baby when there is a mechanical problem. It may be used (rarely in developed countries) in instances of cephalopelvic disproportion or shoulder dystocia when there is no option to perform a caesarean section.

Tachycardia

Tachycardia is a cardiac arrhythmia in which the heart rate becomes abnormally rapid. The incidence of sustained tachycardia in pregnant women is around 2–3 per 1000. Diagnosis is with echocardiography (ECG). Exercise ECG can be reasonably carried out during pregnancy provided that exercise is not contraindicated for obstetric reasons. Drug treatment for pregnant women with supraventricular tachycardia should be administered by experienced medical practitioners in an area with equipment available for resuscitation.

During the initial assessment of a woman in labour, the fetal heart rate should be auscultated (for a minimum of 1 minute immediately after a contraction). A fetal heart rate above 160 beats/min (or below 100 beats/min) should prompt consideration of transfer from midwifery-led to obstetric-led care.

Further reading

Adamson, D.L., Nelson-Piercy, C., 2007. Managing palpitations and arrhythmias during pregnancy. Heart 93(12), 1630–1836. http://www.ncbi.nlm.nih.gov/pmc/articles/PMC2095764/.

National Institute for Health and Care Excellence, 2014. Intrapartum care for healthy women and babies. Clinical guidance 190. https://www.nice.org.uk/guidance/cg190.

Tachypnoea

Tachypnoea in neonates is an abnormal respiratory rate at rest above 60 breaths/min.

It is important to observe the baby's breathing (as part of the initial assessment of the baby's condition after birth and thereafter) when he/she is at rest and when active. The midwife should always start by observing skin colour and then carry out a respiratory inspection, taking into account whether the baby is making either an extra effort or insufficient effort to breathe.

Increased work of breathing

- Tachypnoea is an abnormal respiratory rate at rest above 60 breaths/min.
- Note any inspiratory pulling in of the chest wall above and below the sternum or between the ribs (retraction).
- If nasal flaring is also present, this may indicate that there has been a delay in the lung fluid clearance or that a more serious respiratory problem is developing.
- Grunting, heard either with a stethoscope or audibly, is an abnormal expiratory sound. The grunting baby forcibly exhales against a closed glottis in order to prevent the alveoli from collapsing.

These infants may require help with their breathing, either by intubation or continuous positive airway pressure (CPAP) ventilation.

TENS

Transcutaneous electrical nerve stimulation (TENS) is a method of pain relief involving the use of a mild electrical current. There is insufficient high-quality evidence to support its use as a reliable method of pain relief, although some practitioners have reported that it seems to help some people, depending on the individual and the condition being treated.

Some women have found TENS to be useful in the early stages of labour, but it has not been shown to be effective during the active phase. The National Institute for Health and Care Evidence (NICE) guideline on intrapartum care states that starting to use a TENS machine once the woman is in established labour will not help with pain.

Further reading

NICE, 2014. Intrapartum care for healthy women and babies. Clinical guidance 190. https://www.nice.org.uk/guidance/cg190.

Toxoplasmosis

Toxoplasmosis is caused by *Toxoplasma gondii*, a protozoan parasite found in uncooked meat and cat and dog faeces. Maternal–fetal transmission results from poor hygiene.

Infected neonates may be asymptomatic at birth but can later develop retinal and neurological disease. Babies with subclinical disease can develop seizures, significant cognitive and motor deficits, and reduced cognitive function over time.

Twins

See Multiple pregnancies.

Umbilical cord

The umbilical cord extends from the fetus to the placenta and transmits the umbilical blood vessels, two arteries and one vein. The cord is covered with a layer of amnion continuous with that covering the placenta. The average length of the cord is 50 cm.

Cord blood sampling

This may be required when:

* the mother's blood group is rhesus negative or her rhesus type is unknown
* atypical maternal antibodies have been found during an antenatal screening test
* a haemoglobinopathy is suspected (e.g., sickle cell disease)

The sample should be taken from the fetal surface of the placenta where blood vessels are easily visible.

Cord clamping

After the birth of the baby (or during the birth if the cord is tightly around the baby's neck) the cord is clamped.

Early clamping is carried out in the first 1–3 minutes immediately after birth, regardless of whether cord pulsation has ceased.

Proponents of late clamping suggest that no action be taken until cord pulsation has ceased or the placenta has been delivered.

The optimal time for umbilical cord clamping remains unknown. Delaying cord clamping for at least 2 minutes in a term neonate can be beneficial. A term baby at birth can be drawn up onto the mother's abdomen but raised no higher. A preterm baby should be kept at the level of the placenta to avoid blood draining from the baby to the placenta, resulting in anaemia; if held below the level of the placenta, the baby in effect receives a transfusion.

Further reading

American Congress of Obstetricians and Gynecologists, 2017. Delayed umbilical cord clamping after birth. https://www.acog.org/Resources-And-Publications/Committee-Opinions/Committee-on-Obstetric-Practice/Delayed-Umbilical-Cord-Clamping-After-Birth.

Controlled cord traction

This manoeuvre is believed to reduce blood loss and shorten the third stage of labour, therefore minimizing the time during which the mother is at risk from haemorrhage. It is designed to enhance the normal physiological process. Before starting controlled cord traction (CCT) check that the conditions listed below have been met.

Conditions for starting CCT:

+   a uterotonic drug has been administered
+   it has been given time to act
+   the uterus is well contracted
+   countertraction is applied
+   signs of placental separation and descent are present

At the beginning of the third stage, a strong uterine contraction results in the fundus being palpable below the umbilicus. If tension is applied to the umbilical cord without this contraction, uterine inversion may occur.

When CCT is the preferred method of management, the following sequence of actions is usually undertaken:

+   Once the uterus is found on palpation to be contracted, one hand is placed above the level of the symphysis pubis with the palm facing towards the umbilicus and exerting pressure in an upwards direction. This is countertraction.
+   Grasping the cord, traction is applied in a downward and backward direction following the line of the birth canal.
+   Some resistance may be felt but it is important to apply steady tension by pulling the cord firmly and maintaining the pressure. Jerky movements and force should be avoided.
+   The aim is to complete the action as one continuous, smooth, controlled movement. However, it is only possible to exert this tension for 1 or 2 minutes, as it may be an uncomfortable procedure for the mother and the midwife's hand will tire.
+   Downward traction on the cord must be released *before* uterine countertraction is relaxed, as sudden withdrawal of countertraction while tension is still being applied to the cord may also cause uterine inversion.
+   If the manoeuvre is not immediately successful, there should be a pause before uterine contraction is again checked and a further attempt is made.
+   Should the uterus relax, tension is temporarily released until a good contraction is again palpable.
+   Once the placenta is visible, it may be cupped in the hands to ease pressure on the friable membranes.

- A gentle upward and downward movement or twisting action will help to coax out the membranes and increase the chances of delivering them intact. Great care should be taken to avoid tearing the membranes.

Umbilical haemorrhage

Usually occurs as a result of a poorly applied cord ligature. A purse-string suture should always be inserted if umbilical bleeding does not stop after 15 to 20 minutes.

Umbilical infection

Signs can include localized inflammation and an offensive discharge. Untreated infection can spread to the liver via the umbilical vein and cause hepatitis and septicaemia. Treatment may include:

- regular cleansing
- administration of an antibiotic powder
- appropriate antibiotic therapy

Cord presentation and prolapse

When umbilical cord lies in front of the presenting part, with the fetal membranes still intact, it is termed 'cord presentation'. In cord prolapse, cord lies in front of the presenting part and the fetal membranes are ruptured. When the cord lies alongside, but not in front of, the presenting part, it is described as an occult cord prolapse.

Predisposing factors

Any situation where the presenting part is neither well applied to the lower uterine segment nor well down in the pelvis may make it possible for a loop of cord to slip down in front of the presenting part. Such situations include:

- high or ill-fitting presenting part
- high parity
- prematurity
- malpresentation
- multiple pregnancy
- polyhydramnios

Cord presentation

This is diagnosed on vaginal examination when the cord is felt behind intact membranes. It is, however, rarely detected but may be associated with aberrations in fetal heart monitoring such as decelerations, which occur if the cord becomes compressed.

Management

+ Under no circumstances should the membranes be ruptured.
+ Summon medical aid.
+ Assess fetal wellbeing, using continuous electronic fetal monitoring if available.
+ Help the mother into a position that will reduce the likelihood of cord compression.
+ Caesarean section is the most likely outcome.

Cord prolapse (Fig. 34)

Diagnosis

Diagnosis is made when the cord is felt below or beside the presenting part on vaginal examination. A loop of cord may be visible at the vulva.

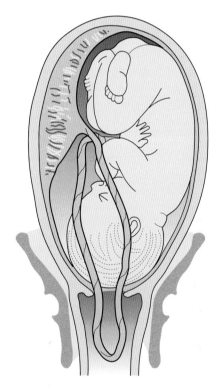

Fig. 34 Cord prolapse.

Whenever there are factors present that predispose to cord prolapse, a vaginal examination should be performed immediately on spontaneous rupture of membranes. Variable decelerations and prolonged decelerations of the fetal heart are associated with cord compression, which may be caused by cord prolapse.

Immediate action and management

Immediate action

+ Call for urgent assistance.
+ If an oxytocin infusion is in progress, this should be stopped.
+ A vaginal examination is performed to assess the degree of cervical dilatation and identify the presenting part and station. If the cord can be felt pulsating, it should be handled as little as possible.
+ If the cord lies outside the vagina, replace it gently to try to maintain temperature.
+ Auscultate the fetal heart rate.
+ Relieve pressure on the cord.
+ Keep your fingers in the woman's vagina and, especially during a contraction, hold the presenting part off the umbilical cord.
+ Help the mother to change position so that her pelvis and buttocks are raised. The knee–chest position causes the fetus to gravitate towards the diaphragm, relieving the compression on the cord.
+ Alternatively, help the mother to lie on her left side, with a wedge or pillow elevating her hips (exaggerated Sims position).
+ The foot of the bed may be raised.
+ These measures need to be maintained until the delivery of the baby, either vaginally or by caesarean section.
+ Consider inserting 500 mL of warm saline into the bladder to relieve the pressure if transfer to an obstetric unit is required.

Treatment

+ Delivery must be expedited with the greatest possible speed.
+ Caesarean section is the treatment of choice if the fetus is still alive and delivery is not imminent or if vaginal birth cannot be indicated.
+ In the second stage of labour the mother may be able to push and you may perform an episiotomy to expedite the birth.
+ Where the presentation is cephalic, assisted birth may be achieved through ventouse or forceps.

Urinary tract infections in newborns

Urinary tract infections can result from bacteria such as *Escherichia coli* or, less often, from a congenital anomaly that obstructs urine flow. The signs are usually those of an early nonspecific infection. Diagnosis is usually confirmed through laboratory evaluation of a urine sample.

Renal/genitourinary system

Urinary infections typically present with lethargy, poor feeding, increasing jaundice and vomiting. Urine that only dribbles out, rather than being passed forcefully, may be an indication of a problem with posterior urethral valves. Urine that is cloudy in appearance or smelly may be an indication of a urinary tract infection.

Renal problems may present as a failure to pass urine. The normal infant usually passes urine 4–10 hours after birth. Normal urine output for a term baby in the first day of life should be 2–4 mL/kg per hour. Urine output of less than 1 mL/kg per hour (oliguria) should be investigated.

Common causes of reduced urine output include:
*   inadequate fluid intake
*   increased fluid loss due to hyperthermia, use of radiant heaters and phototherapy units
*   birth asphyxia
*   congenital abnormalities
*   infection

Uterus

The non-pregnant uterus is a hollow, muscular, pear-shaped organ. It is 7.5 cm long, 5 cm wide and 2.5 cm in depth, each wall being 1.25 cm thick. The cervix forms the lower third of the uterus and measures 2.5 cm in each direction. The uterus consists of the following parts:
*   the body or corpus: this forms the upper two-thirds of the uterus
*   the fundus: the fundus is the domed upper wall between the insertions of the uterine tubes
*   the cornua: these are the upper outer angles of the uterus where the uterine tubes join

The uterine tubes extend laterally from the cornua of the uterus towards the side walls of the pelvis. They arch over the ovaries, the fringed ends hovering near the ovaries in order to receive the ovum. Each tube is 10 cm long. The lumen of the tube provides an open pathway from the outside to the peritoneal cavity. The uterine tube has four portions:
*   the interstitial portion
*   the isthmus
*   the ampulla
*   the infundibulum

The cavity

The cavity is a potential space between the anterior and posterior walls. It is triangular in shape, the base of the triangle being uppermost.

The isthmus

The isthmus is a narrow area between the cavity and the cervix, which is 7 mm long. It enlarges during pregnancy to form the lower uterine segment.

The cervix

This protrudes into the vagina.

- The *internal os* is the narrow opening between the isthmus and the cervix.
- The *external os* is a small round opening at the lower end of the cervix. After childbirth it becomes a transverse slit.
- The *cervical canal* lies between these two ora and is a continuation of the uterine cavity.

Layers

The layers of the uterus are called:

- the endometrium
- the myometrium
- the perimetrium

The endometrium

This forms a lining of ciliated epithelium on a base of connective tissue or stroma.

In the uterine cavity, this endometrium is constantly changing in thickness throughout the menstrual cycle. The basal layer does not alter, but provides the foundation from which the upper layers regenerate. The epithelial cells are cubical in shape and dip down to form glands that secrete an alkaline mucus.

The cervical endometrium does not respond to the hormonal stimuli of the menstrual cycle to the same extent. Here the epithelial cells are tall and columnar in shape and the mucus-secreting glands are branching racemose glands. The cervical endometrium is thinner than that of the body and is folded into a pattern known as the *arbor vitae*. The portion of the cervix that protrudes into the vagina is covered with squamous epithelium similar to that lining the vagina. The point where the epithelium changes, at the external os, is termed the *squamocolumnar junction.*

The myometrium

This layer is thick in the upper part of the uterus but sparser in the isthmus and cervix. Its fibres run in all directions and interlace to surround the blood vessels and lymphatics that pass to and from the endometrium. The outer layer is formed of longitudinal fibres that are continuous with those of the uterine tube, the uterine ligaments and the vagina.

In the cervix the muscle fibres are embedded in collagen fibres, which enable it to stretch in labour.

The perimetrium

This is a double serous membrane, an extension of the peritoneum, which is draped over the uterus, covering all but a narrow strip on either side, and the anterior wall of the supravaginal cervix, from where it is reflected up over the bladder.

Blood supply

The uterine artery arrives at the level of the cervix and is a branch of the internal iliac artery. It sends a small branch to the upper vagina, and then runs upwards in a twisted fashion to meet the ovarian artery and form an anastomosis with it near the cornua. The ovarian artery is a branch of the abdominal aorta. It supplies the ovary and uterine tube before joining the uterine artery. The blood drains through corresponding veins.

Lymphatic drainage

Lymph is drained from the uterine body to the internal iliac glands and also from the cervical area to many other pelvic lymph glands.

Nerve supply

This is mainly from the autonomic nervous system, sympathetic and parasympathetic, via the inferior hypogastric or pelvic plexus.

Physiological changes in pregnancy

The body of the uterus

After conception, the uterus develops to provide a nutritive and protective environment in which the fetus will develop and grow.

Decidua

After embedding of the blastocyst there is thickening and increased vascularity of the lining of the uterus, or decidua. Decidualization, influenced by progesterone and oestradiol, is most marked in the fundus and upper body of the uterus.

+ The decidua is believed to maintain functional quiescence of the uterus during pregnancy; spontaneous labour is thought to result from the activation of the decidua with resultant prostaglandin release following withdrawal of placental hormones.
+ The decidua and trophoblast also produce relaxin, which appears to promote myometrial relaxation, and may have a role to play in cervical ripening and rupture of fetal membranes.

Myometrium

Uterine growth is due to *hyperplasia* (increase in number due to division) and *hypertrophy* (increase in size) of myometrial cells under the influence of oestrogen. The dimensions of the uterus vary considerably, however, depending on the age and parity of the woman.

The three layers of the myometrium become more clearly defined during pregnancy.

Muscle layers

+ The outer longitudinal layer of muscle fibres is thin. It consists of a network of bundles of smooth muscles. These pass longitudinally from the front of the isthmus anteriorly over the fundus and into the vault of the vagina posteriorly, and extend into the round and transverse ligaments.
+ The thicker middle layer comprises interlocked spiral myometrial fibres that are perforated in all directions by blood vessels. Each cell in this layer has a double curve so that the interlacing of any two gives the approximate form of a figure of eight. Due to this arrangement, contraction of these cells after birth causes constriction of the blood vessels, providing 'living ligatures'.
+ The inner circular layer is arranged concentrically around the longitudinal axis of the uterus and bundle formation is diffuse. It forms sphincters around the openings of the uterine tubes and around the internal cervical os.

Uterine activity in pregnancy

The myometrium is both contractile (can lengthen and shorten) and elastic (can enlarge and stretch) to accommodate the growing fetus and allow involution following the birth.

Uterine activity can be measured as early as 7 weeks' gestation, when Braxton Hicks contractions can occur every 20–30 minutes and may reach a pressure of up to 10 mmHg. These contractions facilitate uterine blood flow through the intervillous spaces of the placenta, promoting oxygen delivery to the fetus. Braxton Hicks contractions are usually painless but may cause some discomfort when their intensity exceeds 15 mmHg.

In the last few weeks of pregnancy, *prelabour* occurs:

+ Further increases in myometrial contractions cause the muscle fibres of the fundus to be drawn up.
+ The actively contracting upper uterine segment becomes thicker and shorter in length and exerts a slow, steady pull on the relatively fixed cervix.
+ This causes the beginning of cervical stretching and ripening known as *effacement*, and thinning and stretching of the passive lower uterine segment, but there is no cervical dilatation at this time.

Perimetrium

The perimetrium is a thin layer of peritoneum that protects the uterus. It is deflected over the bladder anteriorly to form the uterovesical pouch, and over the rectum posteriorly to form the pouch of Douglas. The double folds of perimetrium (broad ligaments) become longer and wider with increasing tension exerted on them as the uterus enlarges and rises out of the pelvis.

Blood supply

The uterine blood flow progressively increases from approximately 50 mL/min at 10 weeks' gestation to 450–750 mL/min at term.

Changes in uterine shape and size

For the first few weeks the uterus maintains its original pear shape, but as pregnancy advances the corpus and fundus assume a more globular form (Table 7).

Formation of the upper and lower segments

By the end of pregnancy, the body of the uterus is described as having divided into two anatomically distinct segments.

+ The upper uterine segment is formed from the body of the uterus.
+ The lower uterine segment is formed from the isthmus and the cervix, and is about 8–10 cm in length.

The muscle content reduces from the fundus to the cervix, where it is thinner. When labour begins, the retracted longitudinal fibres in the upper segment pull on the lower segment, causing it to stretch; this is aided by the force applied by the descending presenting part. A ridge forms between the upper and lower uterine segments, known as the *physiological retraction ring*.

Table 7 Changes in the pregnant uterus

10 weeks	The uterus is about the size of an orange
12 weeks	The uterus is about the size of a grapefruit
	It is no longer anteverted and anteflexed and has risen out of the pelvis and become upright
	The fundus may be palpated abdominally above the symphysis pubis
	The globular upper segment is sitting on an elongated stalk formed from the isthmus, which softens and which will treble in length from 7 to 25 mm between the 12th and 36th weeks
20 weeks	The fundus of the uterus can be palpated at the level of the umbilicus
	As the uterus continues to rise in the abdomen, the uterine tubes become progressively more vertical, which causes increasing tension on the broad and round ligaments
30 weeks	The fundus may be palpated midway between the umbilicus and the xiphisternum
38 weeks	The uterus reaches the level of the xiphisternum
	As the upper segment muscle contractions increase in frequency and strength, the lower uterine segment develops more rapidly and is stretched radially; along with cervical effacement and softening of the tissues of the pelvic floor, this permits the fetal presentation to begin its descent into the upper pelvis
	This leads to a reduction in fundal height known as *lightening*, relieving pressure on the upper part of the abdomen but increasing pressure in the pelvis. In the majority of multiparous women, however, engagement rarely occurs prior to labour

Uterus, acute inversion

This is a rare but potentially life-threatening complication of the third stage of labour.

Classification of inversion

Inversion can be classified according to severity as follows:

+ *First-degree.* The fundus reaches the internal os.
+ *Second-degree.* The body or corpus of the uterus is inverted to the internal os (Fig. 35).
+ *Third-degree.* The uterus, cervix and vagina are inverted and are visible.

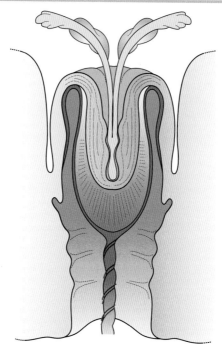

Fig. 35 Second-degree inversion of the uterus.

Causes

Causes of acute inversion are associated with uterine atony and cervical dilatation, and include:

- mismanagement in the third stage of labour, involving excessive cord traction to manage the delivery of the placenta actively
- combining fundal pressure and cord traction to deliver the placenta
- use of fundal pressure while the uterus is atonic, to deliver the placenta
- pathologically adherent placenta
- spontaneous occurrence of unknown cause
- short umbilical cord
- sudden emptying of a distended uterus

Warning signs and diagnosis

- There is haemorrhage, the amount of which will depend on the degree of placental adherence to the uterine wall.

- There is shock and sudden onset of pain.
- The fundus will not be palpable on abdominal examination.
- A mass may be felt on vaginal examination.
- The fundus may be visible at the introitus.

Management
Immediate action

- Summon appropriate medical support.
- Attempt to replace the uterus by pushing the fundus with the palm of the hand, along the direction of the vagina, towards the posterior fornix. The uterus is then lifted towards the umbilicus and returned to position with a steady pressure (Johnson manoeuvre).
- Give hydrostatic pressure with warm saline.
- Insert an intravenous cannula and commence fluids. Take blood for cross-matching prior to starting the infusion.
- If the placenta is still attached, it should be left in situ as attempts to remove it at this stage may result in uncontrollable haemorrhage.
- Once the uterus is repositioned, the operator should keep the hand in situ until a firm contraction is palpated. Oxytocics should be given to maintain the contraction.

Medical management
If manual replacement fails, then medical or surgical intervention is required.

Further reading
Hostetier, D.R., Bosworth, M.F., 2000. Uterine inversion. J. Am. Board Fam. Med. 13 (2), 120–123. http://www.jabfm.org/content/13/2/120.full.pdf+html.
Payne, J., 2015. Uterine inversion. Professional reference. http://patient.info/doctor/uterine-inversion.
Repke, J.T., 2016. Puerperal uterine inversion. http://www.uptodate.com/contents/puerperal-uterine-inversion.

Vaginal birth after caesarean

Planned vaginal birth after caesarean (VBAC) is appropriate for, and may be offered to, the majority of women with a singleton pregnancy with cephalic presentation at 37+ weeks' gestation, who have had a single previous lower segment caesarean delivery, with or without a history of previous vaginal birth. It has a success rate of 72%–75%, but where the woman has experienced previous vaginal birth, particularly VBAC, this increases to 85%–90%.

Successful VBAC has the fewest complications. The greatest risk of adverse outcome is associated with a trial of VBAC resulting in emergency caesarean delivery.

VBAC is contraindicated in women with previous uterine rupture or classical caesarean scar and in women who have other absolute contraindications to vaginal birth that apply, irrespective of the presence or absence of a scar.

An individual assessment of suitability for VBAC should be made in women with factors that increase the risk of uterine rupture. The incidence of uterine rupture in VBAC is 1 in 200 (0.5%).

Planned VBAC should take place in a suitably staffed and equipped delivery suite with resources available for immediate caesarean delivery and advanced neonatal resuscitation.

Further reading

Royal College of Obstetricians and Gynaecologists, 2015. Birth after previous caesarean birth. Green-top guideline no. 45. https://www.rcog.org.uk/globalassets/documents/guidelines/gtg_45.pdf.

White, H.K., le May, A., Cluett, E.R., 2016. Evaluating a midwife-led model of antenatal care for women with a previous caesarean section: a retrospective, comparative cohort study. Birth. Published online 18 Mar 2016. doi: 10.1111/birt.12229. http://onlinelibrary.wiley.com/doi/10.1111/birt.12229/abstract;jsessionid=9ED2B576C80 5FF5A1F0C744AFAC44A2C.f01t03.

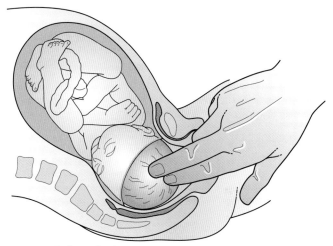

Fig. 36 Vaginal examination.

Vaginal examination

Vaginal examination (Fig. 36) may be carried out to assess progress in labour. Although it is not essential to examine the woman vaginally at frequent intervals, it may be useful to do so when progress is in doubt or another indication arises. Under no circumstances should a midwife make a vaginal examination if there is any frank bleeding, unless the placenta is positively known to be in the upper uterine segment.

The features that are indicative of progress are:

+ effacement and dilatation of the cervix
+ descent, flexion and rotation of the fetal head

Progressive dilatation is monitored as labour continues and charted on either the partograph or the cervicograph.

The level or station of the presenting part is estimated in relation to the ischial spines; during normal labour the head descends progressively. Moulding or a large caput will give a false impression of the level of the fetal head.

In vertex presentations, progress depends partly on increased flexion. Flexion is assessed by the position of the sutures and fontanelles:

+ If the head is fully flexed, the posterior fontanelle becomes almost central.
+ If the head is deflexed, both anterior and posterior fontanelles may be palpable.

Rotation is assessed by noting changes in the position of the fetus between one examination and the next. The sutures and fontanelles are palpated in order to determine position.

Breech presentation

On vaginal examination, the breech feels soft and irregular with no sutures palpable (Fig. 37). The anus may be felt, and fresh meconium on the examining finger is usually diagnostic.

Brow presentation

On vaginal examination, the presenting part is high. The anterior fontanelle may be felt on one side of the pelvis. The orbital ridges and possibly the root of the nose may be felt on the other. A large caput succedaneum may mask these landmarks if the woman has been in labour for some hours.

Face presentation

On vaginal examination, the presenting part is high, soft and irregular (Fig. 38). The orbital ridges, eyes, nose and mouth may be felt. As labour

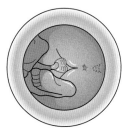

Fig. 37 Feet felt—complete breech presentation.

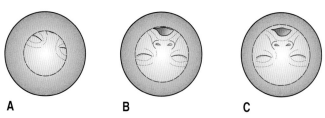

A   **B**   **C**

Fig. 38 Left mentoanterior position. (A) The mentum is felt to the left and anteriorly. (B) Following increased extension of the head, the mouth may be felt. (C) The face has rotated 1/8 circle: orbital ridges in transverse diameter of the pelvis.

progresses the face becomes oedematous, making it more difficult to distinguish from a breech presentation. Care must be taken not to injure or infect the eyes.

Occipitoposterior positions

Findings on vaginal examination will depend on the degree of flexion of the head; locating the anterior fontanelle in the anterior part of the pelvis is diagnostic of occipitoposterior presentation.

Shoulder presentation

Vaginal examination should not be performed without first excluding placenta praevia.

+ In early labour, the presenting part may not be felt.
+ The membranes usually rupture early.
+ If the labour has been in progress for some time, the shoulder may be felt as a soft irregular mass.
+ It is sometimes possible to palpate the ribs, their characteristic grid-iron pattern being diagnostic.
+ When the shoulder enters the pelvic brim, an arm may prolapse; this should be differentiated from a leg.

Vaginal seeding

A process of giving babies born by caesarean section a swab of the mother's vaginal fluids in the belief that it will 'seed' their immune systems to help protect them from developing conditions such as asthma, food allergies and hay fever in later life. The concept has been promoted by advocates of the human microbiome model, who believe that the immune systems of babies born by caesarean section do not develop as fully as if they had been born vaginally. However, maternity staff have been advised against the process, which may carry the risk of infections from exposure to vaginal bacteria; encouraging breast feeding and avoiding unnecessary antibiotics may be more important. Mothers can easily do it themselves, and midwives should respect their autonomy—but should warn them of the potential risks.

Further reading

Cunningham, A., Sim, K., Deieri, A., et al., 2016. "Vaginal seeding" of infants born by caesarean section. Br. Med. J. 352, i227. http://www.bmj.com/content/352/bmj.i227.

Valsalva manoeuvre

The Valsalva manoeuvre describes the process of managed active pushing accompanied by breath holding in the second stage of labour. It is now accepted that this process may have adverse consequences and should not be encouraged.

Varicella zoster

Varicella zoster virus is a highly contagious DNA virus of the herpes family, transmitted by respiratory droplets and contact with vesicle fluid. It causes varicella (chickenpox). The virus has an incubation period of 10–20 days and is infectious from 48 hours before the rash appears until the vesicles crust over.

Maternal deaths have been associated with varicella infection during pregnancy. Effects on the fetus vary with the length of gestation at the time of the infection.

Maternal infection during the first 20 weeks of pregnancy

- There is a 2% risk of fetal varicella syndrome.
- Symptoms can include skin lesions and scarring in a dermatomal distribution, eye problems such as chorioretinitis and cataracts, and skeletal anomalies, in particular limb hypoplasia.
- Severe neurological problems may include encephalitis, microcephaly and significant developmental delay.
- About 30% of babies born with skin lesions die in the first months of life.

Maternal chickenpox from 20 weeks' gestation up to almost the time of birth

- This results in a milder form of neonatal varicella that does not result in negative sequelae for the neonate.

Maternal infection after 36 weeks and particularly in the week before the birth to 2 days after

- Infection rates of up to 50%
- About 25% of those infected will develop neonatal clinical varicella (or varicella infection of the newborn)
- Newborns are also at risk of contracting varicella from mothers or siblings in the postnatal period
- Most affected babies will develop a vesicular rash and about 30% will die
- Other complications of neonatal varicella include clinical sepsis, pneumonia, pyoderma and hepatitis

Ventouse method   See Operative delivery.

Vitamin K deficiency bleeding

Vitamin K deficiency bleeding (VKDB), previously known as *haemorrhagic disease of the newborn*, most commonly occurs between birth and 8 weeks of life, although it may occur up to 12 months. Several proteins—factor II (prothrombin), factor VII (proconvertin), factor IX (plasma thromboplastin component), factor X (thrombokinase) and proteins C and S, require vitamin K for their conversion to active clotting factors. Vitamin K is poorly transferred across the placenta and any stores are quickly depleted after birth. As VKDB is potentially fatal, prophylactic administration of vitamin K is recommended for all newborn babies, either by a single intramuscular injection at birth or, for healthy babies who are not at particular risk of bleeding disorders, orally. Care must be taken to ensure that the appropriate oral regimen is followed as more than one oral dose is required.

Further reading

British National Formulary for Children: Vitamin K deficiency bleeding. https://bnfc.nice.org.uk/treatment-summary/vitamins.html.

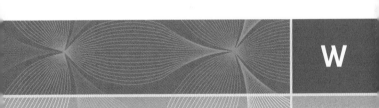

Water birth

Therapeutic use of water in childbirth has grown in popularity, and most maternity units now offer a birthing pool. Some women may wish to spend most of their labour and birth in the water pool, others choose to spend short periods and some women may wish to leave the water for the actual birth of the baby and delivery of the placenta. There is evidence for a number of benefits to labouring in water, particularly a reduced need for pharmacological analgesia, but the midwife should determine the benefits and risks for each woman.

Essential considerations include:

Temperature of the water

+ Too high a temperature will be uncomfortable for the woman and may cause fetal tachycardia.
+ Cooler temperatures may induce respiration before the baby has been brought to the surface.

Time of entry to water

+ Immersion in water in the early stages of labour may inhibit uterine activity. Some midwives recommend delaying entering the water until the cervix is 4–5 cm dilated, although there is little research to support or refute this practice.

Infection of mother or baby

+ Infection risk appears to be very low and can be minimized by using disposable bath linings where available, and by thorough cleaning of the bath after use in line with infection control policies.

Water embolism

+ In theory, water may enter the maternal circulation via the placental bed, causing a water embolism. It is recommended that the third stage of labour should be conducted out of the water. Oxytocic drugs (if used) should be given when the woman has left the water.

Perineal trauma

+ The midwife should provide verbal support to enable the woman to control the birth and allow the head and shoulders to emerge slowly, to minimize the risk of perineal trauma.

Monitoring maternal and fetal health

+ Auscultate the fetal heart using an underwater ultrasonic monitor, wireless electronic fetal monitoring or Pinard stethoscope.
+ Inhalation analgesia is suitable if pain relief is required. Do not leave the woman unattended.
+ If narcotic analgesia is required, the woman should be asked to leave the water, as the drowsiness induced by the drugs may compromise safety.

The baby

The baby should be brought to the surface immediately after birth. The umbilical cord should not be clamped and cut while the baby is still under the water as the sudden reduction in placental–fetal blood flow may initiate respiration and, therefore, inspiration of water. If the umbilical cord needs to be cut prior to the birth of the baby, the woman should be asked to stand with the baby's head clear of the water so that cord may be clamped and cut before the birth of the shoulders.

Weight gain in pregnancy

Average weight gain during pregnancy is about 12.5 kg; however, this varies according to the woman's pre-pregnancy body mass index (BMI). BMI = weight in kilograms/square of the height in metres (Table 8). Those with a low BMI are expected to gain more weight, whereas women who are obese should gain less.

Table 8 **Classification of body mass index**

Category	Pre-pregnant BMI (kg/m²)
Low (underweight)	<18.5
Normal	18.5–24.9
High (overweight)	25.0–29.9
Obese	>29.9

Wharton jelly

Wharton jelly is a gelatinous substance that provides insulation and protection of the blood vessels within the umbilical cord against extension, bending, twisting and compression. It is a primitive connective tissue (primary mesenchyme) and contains stem cells (in addition to those present in umbilical cord blood) as well as lipids and growth factors.

Woods manoeuvre

Woods manoeuvre (Fig. 39) is used to assist in the delivery of the baby in shoulder dystocia. The woman should be assisted into the lithotomy position or onto all fours to remove restrictions to the sacrum and coccyx (present when the mother is in the dorsal or semirecumbent position). The midwife applies one hand to the mother's abdomen, putting firm but gentle pressure onto the fetal buttocks, and inserts the other into the vagina to locate the anterior surface of the posterior shoulder (clavicle). The shoulder is then rotated through 180 degrees in the direction of the fetal back, which causes an abduction of the fetal shoulders. This rotation may dislodge the anterior shoulder and enable the posterior shoulder to enter the pelvic brim. The shoulders may then be delivered by normal downward traction and the delivery completed.

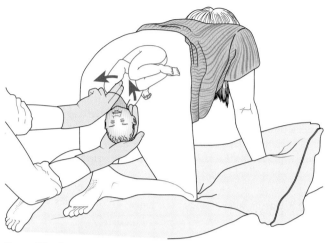

Fig. 39 **Woods manoeuvre.**

Z

Zavanelli manoeuvre

A manoeuvre of last resort in the management of shoulder dystocia, in which the fetal head is manually flexed and returned to the vagina prior to delivery being undertaken by caesarean section.

Zika virus

Zika virus is a mosquito-borne infection which has been associated with profound effects on the unborn fetus in pregnant women. It was first reported in Africa in the 1940s, but few outbreaks have been documented prior to the major outbreak in Brazil in 2015. It has since spread rapidly over most countries in South and Central America and the Caribbean.

The majority of people infected with Zika virus have no symptoms but, where they occur, they include rash, itching/pruritis, fever, headache, arthralgia and myalgia. The illness tends to be mild and self-limiting within 2–7 days.

The major concern is that Zika virus is a cause of microcephaly and other congenital anomalies (congenital Zika syndrome). Zika can cross the placental barrier, and it is likely that infection in early pregnancy poses the greatest risk.

Pregnant women who have recently travelled in an area reporting active Zika virus transmission in the last 9 months should seek advice from their midwife on their return to the UK, even if they have not been unwell. A detailed travel history should be undertaken.

Testing for the virus is by reverse transcription polymerase chain reaction on a maternal blood sample. The test may also be performed on a sample of amniotic fluid, after careful assessment of the risk of miscarriage or preterm birth, although it is not known how sensitive this test is for congenital infection or the likelihood of an infected fetus subsequently developing a fetal abnormality.

Where the virus is detected on laboratory testing, the woman should be referred to a fetal medicine service for further assessment. If the test result is negative, serial (4-weekly) fetal ultrasound scans should be considered to monitor fetal growth and anatomy. If a significant brain abnormality or microcephaly is confirmed (by magnetic resonance imaging of the fetal brain) the option of termination of pregnancy should be discussed with the woman, regardless of gestation.

Following birth

Following a live birth where there has been laboratory confirmation of maternal or fetal Zika virus infection, the following tests are recommended:

- histopathological examination of the placenta and umbilical cord
- testing of placental tissue and cord tissue for Zika virus RNA
- testing of cord blood and neonatal urine for Zika virus and other flaviviruses

If congenital infection is subsequently confirmed, the baby should be followed up into childhood for signs of any adverse sequelae.

Further reading

National Travel Health Network and Centre (NaTHNac), 2017. Zika virus – update and advice for travellers. https://travelhealthpro. org.uk/news/4/zika-virus-update-and-advice-for-travellers.

Continued

Further reading—cont'd

Public Health England, 2017. Zika virus: algorithm for assessing pregnant women with a history of travel during pregnancy https://www.gov.uk/government/uploads/system/uploads/attachment_data/file/634373/.

Royal College of Midwives, 2016. The latest Zika virus advice for March. https://www.rcm.org.uk/news-views-and-analysis/news/the-latest-zika-virus-advice-for-march.

Royal College of Obstetricians and Gynaecologists, Royal College of Midwives, Public Health England, Health Protection Scotland, 2016 (Updated July 2017). Interim RCOG/RCM/PHE/HPS clinical guidelines: Zika virus infection and pregnancy. Information for healthcare professionals. https://www.rcog.org.uk/globalassets/documents/news/zika-virus-rcog-july-2017.pdf.